Management of Zenker and Hypopharyngeal Diverticula

Richard Scher • David Myssiorek
Editors

Management of Zenker and Hypopharyngeal Diverticula

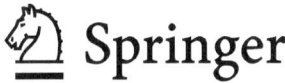 Springer

Editors
Richard Scher
ENT Procedure Innovation
and Development
Olympus Corporation of the Americas
Southborough, MA
USA

David Myssiorek
Otolaryngology
Jacobi Medical Center
Department of Surgery
Bronx, NY
USA

ISBN 978-3-319-92155-6   ISBN 978-3-319-92156-3   (eBook)
https://doi.org/10.1007/978-3-319-92156-3

Library of Congress Control Number: 2018950454

Printed on acid-free paper

This Springer imprint is published by Springer Nature, under the registered company Springer International Publishing AG
The registered company address is: Gewerbestrasse 11, 6330 Cham, Switzerland

Preface

Normal swallowing is essential to the maintenance of physical and psychological health. Anything that disrupts the ability to swallow may compromise nutrition and adversely impact social interaction and enjoyment, ultimately leading to diminished overall quality of life and life expectancy.

Of the myriad disorders that cause dysphagia, Zenker diverticula (ZD) and other hypopharyngeal diverticula represent a unique set of pathologies that adversely impact individuals. Although relatively uncommon in the overall population, ZD and hypopharyngeal diverticula can have a profound impact on the ability to eat and maintain adequate nutrition needed for good health.

It is remarkable how the evolution of treatment of these diverticula has progressed. Numerous luminaries within the fields of otolaryngology, surgery, and gastroenterology have contributed to the medical knowledge base of these disorders and the development of effective treatment approaches. Names such as Friedrich Albert von Zenker, Charles Bell (of Bell's palsy notoriety), Gustav Killian, Emil Kocher, Frank Lahey, Harris Mosher, and Gustav Dohlman have all contributed to these advancements.

Over the past century, significant medical advances have occurred allowing patients with diverticula to receive more effective and safe treatment [1]. These treatments have resulted in resolution of the deleterious health effects seen with these conditions, with recent surgical innovations reducing the impact of treatment on patients with ZD and other hypopharyngeal diverticula. These newer, minimally invasive surgical treatment approaches have made treatment safer and more effective [2].

ZD and hypopharyngeal diverticula overwhelmingly affect older individuals. Frequently, these people have additional comorbidities. In the United States, the number of people older than 65 years will increase from 35.6 million in the year 2000 to 70 million by the year 2030. By the year 2050, 20% of the population will be over 65 with 20 million over the age of 85 [3]. Worldwide, there were 600 million people over the age of 60 in the year 2000. By 2025, that number will increase to 1.2 billion, and it is expected to rise to two billion by 2050 [4]. The incidence of ZD is estimated to be 2/100,000 in the United States [5]. This number is likely larger because smaller diverticula are often not reported due to lack of specific symptomatology. As our population ages, the techniques used to diagnose and treat ZD will likely become more and more significant.

It is our intention that this book will serve as a definitive resource for surgeons and clinicians responsible for the evaluation and care of patients with ZD and hypopharyngeal diverticula. Approaches to the anatomy, physiology, and the factors leading to the development of a hypopharyngeal diverticulum are presented. Methods of diagnosing and evaluating hypopharyngeal diverticula will also be discussed. The book reviews the surgical approaches used historically as a context for an in-depth discussion and presentation of newer, less invasive endoscopic approaches for therapy. The surgical techniques used with these endoscopic approaches, and the technological advances that have made them possible, will be presented in detail along with the results, indications, limitations, and alternatives to these treatments.

Expected clinical outcomes with these approaches will be contrasted with alternative, more invasive surgical techniques that remain useful in select situations. Detailed information on these more invasive techniques will be presented as well, in order that the text serve as a comprehensive resource to all surgeons and clinicians who may still occasionally have need for these treatment approaches. Newer, more novel investigational treatment approaches, including flexible endoscopic therapy, will be presented and discussed to provide up-to-date information and data for clinicians and surgeons.

The textbook will serve as a resource for surgeons, physicians, other clinicians, and students dealing with and learning about ZD and hypopharyngeal diverticula. The information will be comprehensively covered with the intent to provide a primary source of clinical information useful to those caring for these patients. The textbook chapters will be written by experts on these topics, with contributors representing the specialties of otolaryngology—head and neck surgery, gastroenterology, radiology, and speech and swallowing sciences.

We hope the readers of this book will enjoy the content and find it informative and supportive as they manage patients with ZD and hypopharyngeal diverticula. Perhaps it will encourage further discovery into the diagnosis and treatment of these diverticula. As the last century saw great strides in improving the care and outcome for patients with these disorders, perhaps the next 100 years will lead to even greater therapeutic outcomes as a result of the development and adoption of more advanced technology.

References

1. Hillel AT, Flint PW. Evolution of endoscopic surgical therapy for Zenker's diverticulum. Laryngoscope. 2009;119:39–44.
2. Wilken R, Whited C, Scher RL. Endoscopic staple diverticulostomy for Zenker's diverticulum. Review of experience in 337 cases. Ann Otol Rhinol Laryngol. 2015;124:21–9.
3. Department of Health and Human Services. A profile of older Americans: 2011. Available at: http://www.aoa.gov/Aging_Statistics/Profile/2011/docs/2011profile.pdf.

4. Gervasi R, Orlando G, Lerose MA, Amato B, Docimo G, Zeppa P, Puzziello A. Thyroid surgery in geriatric patients: a literature review. BMC Surg. 2012;12 Suppl 1:S16.
5. Achem SR, DeVault KR. Dysphagia in aging. J Clin Gastroenterol. 2005;39:357–71.

Southborough, MA, USA   Richard L. Scher
Bronx, NY, USA   David Myssiorek

Acknowledgements

It has been a great honor, and a genuine learning experience, to have some of the leading clinicians caring for patients with swallowing disorders participate in the preparation of this textbook detailing the management of patients with Zenker and other hypopharyngeal diverticula. This text and its contents represents a step in a journey that started over 25 years ago, when I had the great fortune to train with and observe Haskins (Chuck) Kashima, MD, treat patients with Zenker diverticula using an endoscopic laser technique. This was revelatory, as I had previously been exclusively trained to perform external diverticulectomy and cricopharyngeal myotomy by outstanding surgeons who genuinely believed that endoscopic approaches were too often associated with complications and far too risky for a patient population that was most often elderly and infirm. Dr. Kashima's approach was meticulous and exacting, and led to excellent outcomes for his patients, but not without some clinical concerns postoperatively that often required several days in hospital. This encouraged me and William J. Richtsmeier, MD, PhD, a mentor, friend, and contributor to this textbook, to think about ways that endoscopic treatment could be done more safely, without compromising effectiveness for relief of dysphagia. The result of our collaboration, along with the efforts of other clinicians worldwide, led to the widespread adoption of endoscopic staple diverticulostomy (ESD) as a leading treatment for patients with Zenker diverticulum. Over the ensuing 20 years others have advanced treatment by this and other endoscopic approaches, with continually improved patient outcomes reported.

Our efforts to help patients with Zenker and other hypopharyngeal diverticula would not have been possible without the first patient who agreed to undergo ESD, a new and still unproven treatment. I have never forgotten the trust he placed in me to fulfill his desire to have his symptoms relieved without a major surgical procedure. Similarly, I am forever grateful to the many patients with diverticula who came to see me, often from great distances, who offered me the opportunity to provide their care. To my colleagues at Duke University who supported my care of patients with Zenker diverticulum and were willing to defer their own involvement in treatment, I can only say thank you. In creating an environment in which our patients received the highest level of care and I was able to constantly strive to improve patient outcomes, perhaps no one was more responsible than Kitty Lockner, RN. She is truly an angel in white, and my gratitude for her support and assistance is immense.

The interest, support, and love of my family have been invaluable. They have always been willing to hear about what I was doing for patients with "bags" in their throats, and their fascination helped to keep mine fresh. Finally, my partner, Doris Iarovici, MD, has been a constant source of support and a sounding board for all my professional efforts. It was a joy to share my last procedure in practice, treatment of a patient with Zenker diverticulum by ESD, with her, and a moment I will long remember.

On behalf of David Myssiorek and me, a sincere thank you to Dhanapal Palanisamy, Project Coordinator at Springer, for guiding us through the process of organizing this book and for constant positive reminders that helped us and all the authors complete our work as efficiently as possible. Our appreciation extends to Samantha Lonuzzi, Assistant Editor, and Springer, for deciding to support us in this project, and for believing in the need for a textbook to help educate and guide clinicians caring for patients with Zenker and other hypopharyngeal diverticula.

Lastly, my thanks to coeditor David Myssiorek, MD, for his efforts to make this textbook outstanding and for his constant belief in me. His encouragement and insistence that we share our experience in treating patients with diverticula has been a major factor in undertaking and completing this project. Through it all he has been a supportive colleague and friend.

Richard L. Scher

I became extremely interested in hypopharyngeal diverticula after treating a patient and having more than one serious complication. At the time, I had contacted Dr. Scher to speak at a regional meeting regarding his endoscopic technique. I was so impressed by his presentation that I was encouraged by my Chairman, Dr. Allan Abramson, to start a program at our institution. Dr. Scher and I arranged for me to observe him performing two endoscopic staple diverticulotomies. That day changed my view on the treatment and care of these patients. For this, I am eternally grateful to my coeditor.

In the composition of this book, we discovered the rich history involved with this peculiar disorder. Many famous men (and women) were involved in the evolution of its treatment. The modern version of the Hippocratic Oath contains this pledge: "I will respect the hard-won scientific gains of those physicians in whose steps I walk, and gladly share such knowledge as is mine with those who are to follow." It is our hope that we have lived up to our obligation to the Oath. Combined, the editors of this book have had the honor of training hundreds of medical students, interns, residents, and fellows in our field. Bringing advances in medicine and surgery to these young women and men is richly rewarding. Much of what was written in this book stems from original research and lectures delivered to our pupils, and for this, we are grateful to be able to pass on this knowledge.

David Myssiorek

Contents

Contributors

Todd H. Baron, MD, FASGE Division of Gastroenterology and Hepatology, University of North Carolina, Chapel Hill, NC, USA

Hayley Born, MD Department of Otolaryngology, University of Cincinnati, Cincinnati, OH, USA

C. Scott Brown, MD Division of Head and Neck Surgery and Communication Sciences, Department of Surgery, Duke University Medical Center, Durham, NC, USA

Keith A. Chadwick, MD Department of Otolaryngology—Head and Neck Surgery, Oregon Health and Science University, Portland, OR, USA

Seth M. Cohen, MD, MPH Division of Head and Neck Surgery and Communication Sciences, Department of Surgery, Duke University Medical Center, Durham, NC, USA

Mark A. Fritz, MD Department of Otolaryngology—Head and Neck Surgery, University of Kentucky, Lexington, KY, USA

Rebecca J. Howell, MD Department of Otolaryngology, University of Cincinnati, Cincinnati, OH, USA

Christopher M. Johnson, MD Department of Otolaryngology, Naval Medical Center, San Diego, CA, USA

Tawfiq Khoury, MD Division of Head and Neck Surgery and Communication Sciences, Department of Surgery, Duke University Medical Center, Durham, NC, USA

Natalie A. Krane, MD Department of Otolaryngology—Head and Neck Surgery, Oregon Health and Science University, Portland, OR, USA

Ryan Law, DO Division of Gastroenterology and Hepatology, University of Michigan, Ann Arbor, MI, USA

Albert L. Merati, MD, FACS Department of Otolaryngology—Head and Neck Surgery, University of Washington School of Medicine, Seattle, WA, USA

David Myssiorek, MD, FACS Jacobi Medical Center, Bronx, NY, USA

Department of Otolaryngology, Albert Einstein College of Medicine, Bronx, NY, USA

Molly Naunheim, MD Department of Otolaryngology—Head and Neck Surgery, University of California—San Francisco, San Francisco, CA, USA

Gregory N. Postma, MD Department of Otolaryngology—Head and Neck Surgery, Medical College of Georgia at Augusta University, Augusta, GA, USA

William J. Richtsmeier, MD, PhD, FACS Division of Otolaryngology, Bassett Medical Center, Cooperstown, NY, USA

Richard L. Scher, MD, FACS ENT Procedure Innovation and Development, Olympus Corporation, Tokyo, Japan,

Division of Head and Neck Surgery and Communication Sciences, Department of Surgery, Duke University, Durham, NC, USA

Joshua S. Schindler, MD Department of Otolaryngology—Head and Neck Surgery, Oregon Health and Science University, Portland, OR, USA

Philip A. Weissbrod, MD Division of Otolaryngology—Head and Neck Surgery, Department of Surgery, University of California San Diego, La Jolla, CA, USA

Laurie Wennerholm, MA, CCC-SLP, BCS-S Speech Pathology and Swallowing Center for Cancer Care, White Plains Hospital/Montefiore Health System, White Plains, NY, USA

The History of Zenker Diverticulum and Its Treatment

Richard L. Scher and David Myssiorek

Although named after Friedrich Albert von Zenker (Fig. 1.1), the Zenker diverticulum (ZD) was actually first described by Abraham Ludlow in 1769 [1]. This was followed by case reports from Italy and Germany later in the same century [2]. As many as 20 reports preceded Zenker's description in 1877.

Hugo von Ziemssen, a professor in the Department of Medicine, joined Zenker in publishing *Krankheiten des Oesophagus* in which they reported 34 patients with these outpouchings and correctly postulated that these were pulsion diverticula [3].

Before von Zenker's work, there were some elaborate theories about the cause of these rare entities. In Ludlow's original description of hypopharyngeal diverticula, he described finding a cherry pit in the sac and hypothesized it to be the source of the sac. Pepper, bread, bones, and lead shot were reported as possible etiologies by other authors [4]. Westrin [4] cited Fridberg regarding an officer who struck his head and neck and developed neck swelling. Within a year, the officer was found to have a diverticulum and died of starvation. Fridberg thought this was secondary to a ruptured constrictor. Another report of a burn in the throat resulting in a diverticulum was published. More fanciful etiologic theories existed as well, such as compression of the larynx by goiter and tight shirt collars [4]. The attribution of the hypopharyngeal diverticulum to Zenker resulted because of his systematic study of these anomalies and a description of their causation resulting from altered intraluminal pressure dynamics.

R. L. Scher (✉)
ENT Procedure Innovation and Development, Olympus Corporation, Tokyo, Japan

Division of Head and Neck Surgery and Communication Sciences, Department of Surgery, Duke University, Durham, NC, USA
e-mail: richard.scher@olympus.com

D. Myssiorek
Jacobi Medical Center, Bronx, NY, USA
Department of Otolaryngology, Albert Einstein College of Medicine, Bronx, NY, USA

© Springer International Publishing AG, part of Springer Nature 2018
R. Scher, D. Myssiorek (eds.), *Management of Zenker and Hypopharyngeal Diverticula*, https://doi.org/10.1007/978-3-319-92156-3_1

Fig. 1.1 Friedrich Albert
von Zenker. https://en.
wikipedia.org/wiki/
Friedrich_Albert_von_
Zenker

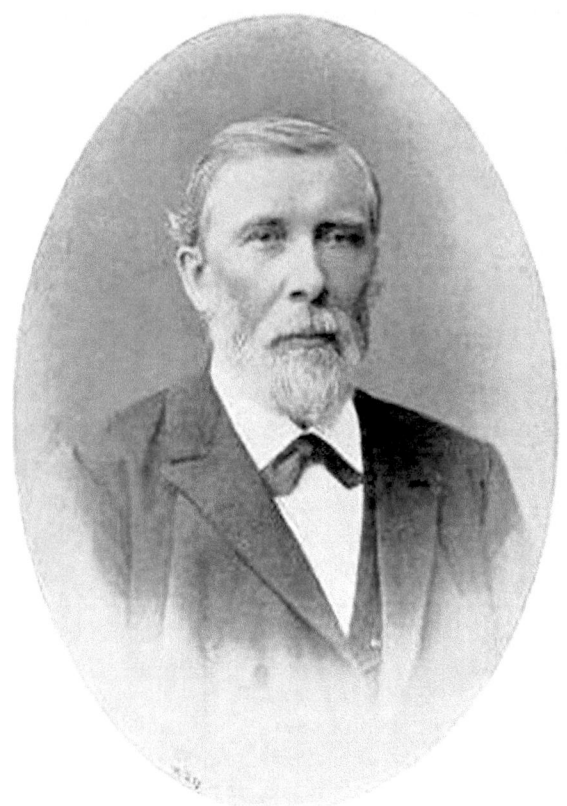

The more modern theory of ZD formation requires two factors: muscular hypertonicity of the cricopharyngeus muscle and a weakness in the posterior pharyngeal wall. Sir Charles Bell first described this as the etiology of ZD in 1816 [5]. In 1908, the anatomical weakness between the inferior constrictor muscle and the cricopharyngeus was described by Killian [6]. Several theories about genesis of ZD were promoted which will be covered in the physiology chapter of this book. Currently, many authors support the theory that despite normal relaxation, the cricopharyngeus does not fully open. Frequent increased luminal pressure and a weakened hypopharyngeal region allow for herniation of mucosa. ZD, as a pulsion diverticulum, is not covered in muscle. There is evidence that the cricopharyngeus muscle is inflamed and fibrotic in specimens taken during surgery [7].

As a result of recognizing the serious sequelae of malnutrition and aspiration associated with ZD, various treatment approaches were attempted. Originally Zenker recommended serial dilation of the upper esophageal sphincter [3]. Bell advanced draining of the pouch by cutaneous fistulization [5]. The first successful external ZD excision was performed by Wheeler in 1885 [8]. Kocher performed diverticulum excision and primary wound closure 7 years later [9]. Girard described invaginating the diverticulum and then oversewing it in 1896, but the recurrence rate was high and the procedure was abandoned [10]. Goldmann performed a two-step approach to diverticulum excision [11]. The diverticular sac was ligated at its neck, and the distal sac was brought out externally to the wound. The wound was packed and closed within 2 months. This was modified and championed by Lahey, who in 1954 reported reasonable results in 365 patients [12]. This was one of the first descriptions advocating for inclusion of myotomy of the cricopharyngeus muscle in the treatment scheme for all patients undergoing surgery. However, ZD tend to occur in older individuals, and baseline diminished health made two operations difficult to tolerate. Gradually a one-stage excision became more popular as improved anesthesia and antibiotics lowered the reported mortality rate of ZD excision to close to 1%.

In 1912, Schmid advanced diverticulopexy by suspending the distal pouch high in the neck, thus alleviating food collection in the sac [13]. In 1899, Richardson performed the first reported cricopharyngeal myotomy [14]. Aubin was the first to propose cricopharyngeal myotomy as a useful adjunct to open diverticulectomy [15]. Harrison promoted cricopharyngeal myotomy for ZD in 1958 [16]. More recently, cricopharyngeal myotomy alone has become a reasonable solution for select patients.

During the first half of the twentieth century, surgeons started to excise the sac and close the wound during one procedure. This was not done earlier due to catastrophic complications such as fistula, mediastinitis, and death. In 1965, Payne and Clagett reported the results of 478 patients operated with a single-stage diverticulum excision with a reduced rate of complications compared to historical results [17]. However, without treatment of the cricopharyngeal muscle, the pathophysiologic mechanism that created not only the diverticulum but the dysphagia symptoms remained intact. Recurrence was not uncommon. As early as 1966, one author maintained that ZD excision without cricopharyngeal myotomy would fail [18]. In 1962 Sutherland promoted cricopharyngeal myotomy alone for ZD [19]. Since that time, cricopharyngeal myotomy has been advocated as part of all operations for ZD.

An endoscopic approach to treat ZD by dividing the cricopharyngeal muscle was first attempted by Mosher [20] (Fig. 1.2). He divided the common wall between the diverticulum and esophagus with a knife. Six out of seven patients succeeded, but one died. Seiffert was endoscopically dividing the common wall using a pair of scissors [21]. However, these procedures were fraught with the development of mediastinitis and high mortality rates. This set the stage for Gosta Dohlman, professor of otorhinolaryngology at Lund University in Sweden (Fig. 1.3). Dohlman and Mattsson published their paper on 100 patients treated endoscopically whose common wall was divided with diathermic electrocautery [22]. The reported success rate was 93%. They modified a rigid esophagoscope to allow adequate exposure of the common wall between the ZD and esophagus in order to accomplish the surgical goal. They reported no significant complications, although subsequent authors could not reproduce their low complication rate and continued to have mediastinitis occur frequently.

Fig. 1.2 Harris P. Mosher, MD

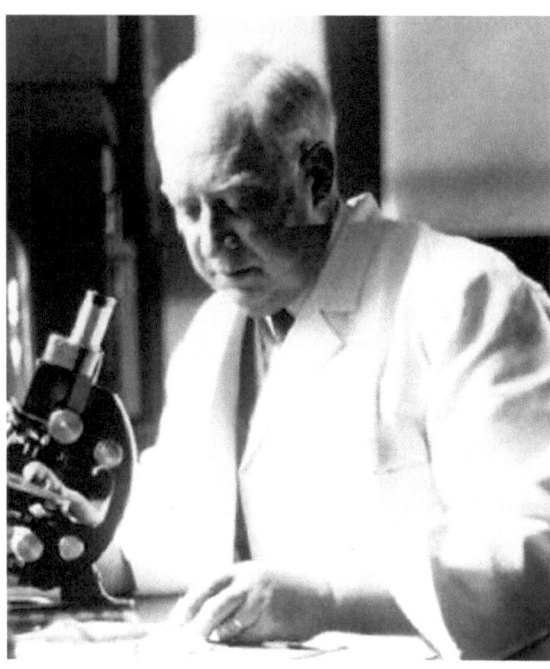

Fig. 1.3 Gosta Dohlman, Professor of Otorhinolaryngology at Lund University. http://www. medicinhistoriskasyd.se/ smhs_bilder/displayimage. php?album=10&pid=900

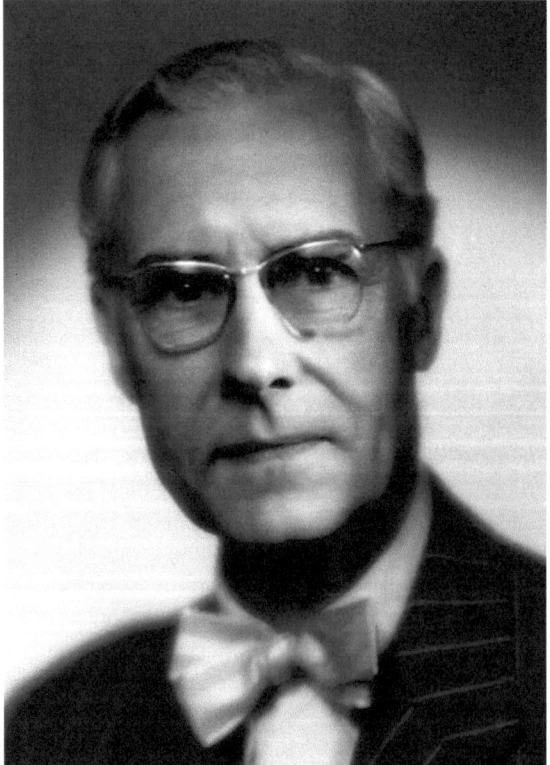

The high complication rate associated with the Dohlman procedure resulted in its lack of popularity and adoption. Operating microscopes, fiber-optic telescopes, and newer surgical tools sparked new interest in treating ZD with endoscopic surgery. Among the tools introduced to divide the common wall were CO_2 lasers, KTP lasers, papillotomes, and argon beam coagulation [2]. In 1978, Weerda introduced a distending laryngoscope and modified it in 1981 by extending the blade to 24 cm [23] (Fig. 1.4). This allowed improved access to the esophageal introitus. Other access methods followed, including the use of Feyh-Kastenbauer suspension retractors (Gyrus ACMI (www.gyrus-ent.com)/Explorent GmbH, Tuttlingen, Germany). These instruments allowed relatively wide access to both the esophagus and mouth of the diverticulum. In turn, this allowed the application of lasers, staplers, and other power devices to divide the common wall during endoscopic exposure.

The latest additions to the endoscopic surgical armamentarium were linear staplers. The use of staplers in conjunction with endoscopic treatment of ZD was first reported in Belgium by Collard's group and Martin Hirsch in England, both in 1993 [24, 25]. The dual benefits of hemostasis and decreased incidence of mediastinitis were immediately apparent. Ultimately, Scher and Richtsmeier published a series of six patients operated in the United States in 1996 ushering in the popularized use of endoscopic staple-assisted diverticulostomy [26]. The advantages of reduced surgical morbidity coupled with rapid convalescence quickly made the endoscopic staple diverticulostomy the procedure of choice for treatment of patients with ZD.

Further advances in endoscopic treatment for ZD using flexible endoscopic approaches have been reported. In 1995, Mulder and Ishioka independently described the use and perceived benefits of using flexible endoscopic guidance to

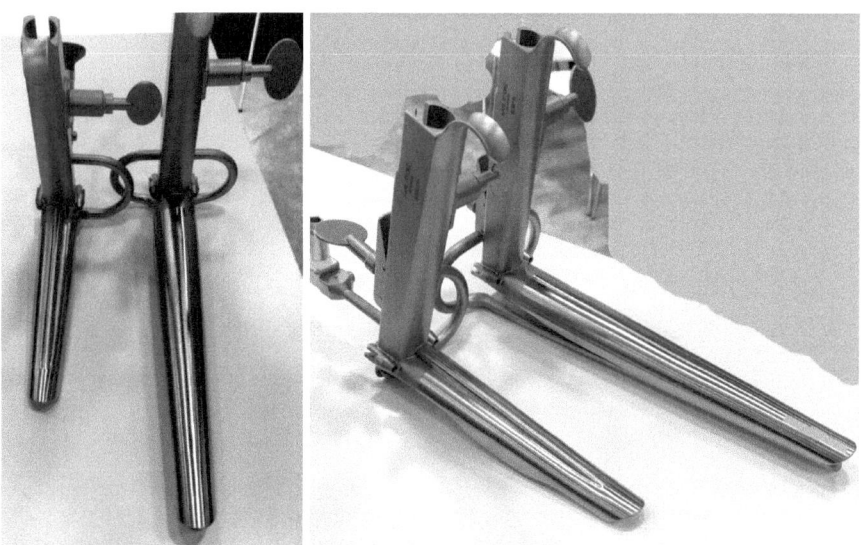

Fig. 1.4 Weerda bivalve distending laryngoscope and diverticuloscope

divide the diverticular common wall [27, 28]. Since then many reports have provided some evidence of the applicability of this approach, with the proposed benefits being no requirement for general anesthesia, no need for neck extension, and good relief of symptoms [29, 30]. This approach may require more than one treatment for each patient in order to achieve success and, in practice, often has required patient sedation for tolerance.

Conclusion

From Zenker's description and etiologic theory to Mosher's ingenuity and Dohlman and Mattson's perseverance, to Collard and Martin Hirsch's creativity and problem-solving, the diagnosis and treatment of ZD have advanced significantly over the past 140 years. In large part, current treatment approaches have been made possible by technologic advancements and application that have allowed surgeons to refine treatment into a less invasive and morbid experience for patients with ZD. As subsequent chapters in this text will demonstrate, current perioperative care regimens have now broadened the surgical armamentarium to allow safe and effective treatments for ZD using both endoscopic and open approaches, allowing physicians to choose the optimum method tailored to the patient's individual need. It is likely that further advances and study will lead to even greater improvements in treatment for ZD over the next 100 years.

References

1. Ludlow A. A case of obstructed deglutition from a preternatural dilatation of and bag formed in the pharynx. Med Observ Inq. 1769;3:85–101.
2. Stewart K, Sen P. Pharyngeal pouch management: an historical review. J Laryngol Otol. 2016;130(2):116–20.
3. Zenker FA, von Ziemssen H. Diseases of the esophagus. In: Von Ziemssen H, editor. Handbook of special pathology and therapy [in German], vol. 7. Leipzig: FCW Vogel; 1877.
4. Westrin KM, Ergün S, Carlsöö B. Zenker's diverticulum--a historical review and trends in therapy. Acta Otolaryngol. 1996;116(3):351–60.
5. Bell C. Surgical observations. London: Longmans, Greene and Co; 1816. p. 64–70.
6. Killian G. The leader of the oesophagus. Ann Mal Oreille Larynx. 1908;34:1.
7. Cook IJ, Blumbergs P, Cash K, Jamieson GG, Shearman DJ. Structural abnormalities of the cricopharyngeal muscle in patients with Zenker diverticulum. J Gastroenterol Hepat. 1992;7:556–62.
8. Gregoire J, Duranceau A. Surgical management of Zenker's diverticulum. Hepatogastroenterology. 1992;39:132–8.
9. Kocher T. The oesophageal diverticulum and its treatment [in German]. Cor-BI f Schweiz Aerzite. 1892;22:233–44.
10. Girard C. The treatment of oesophageal diverticulae [in French]. Congress Fr Chir. 1896;10:392–407.
11. Goldmann EE. The two sided operation of pulsion diverticula of the oesophagus: in addition to remarks on the esophageal opening [in German]. Beitr Klin Chir. 1909;61:741–9.
12. Lahey FH, Warren KW. Esophageal diverticula. Surg Gynecol Obstet. 1954;98:1–28.

13. Schmid HH. Proposal of a simple procedure for treating oesophageal diverticula [in German]. Wien Klin Wochenschr. 1912;25:487–8.
14. Richardson M. Two cases of oesophageal diverticulum, with remarks. Ann Surg. 1900;31:525.
15. Aubin A. Un cas de diverticule de pulsion de l'oesophage traite par la resection de la poche associee a l'oesophagotomie extramuqueuse. Ann d'Otolaryngol. 1936;2:167–77.
16. Harrison MS. The aetiology, diagnosis and surgical treatment of pharyngeal diverticula. J Laryngol Otol. 1958;72:523–34.
17. Payne WS, Clagett OT. Pharyngeal and esophageal diverticula. Curr Probl Surg. 1965;2:1–31.
18. Belsey R. Functional disease of the esophagus. J Thorac Cardiovasc Surg. 1966;52:164–88.
19. Sutherland HD. Cricopharyngeal achalasia. J Thorac Cardiovasc Surg. 1962;43:114–26.
20. Mosher HP. Webs and pouches of the esophagus, their diagnosis and treatment. Surg Gynecol Obstet. 1917;25:175–87.
21. Seiffert A. Oesophagoskopie und endoskopische Oesophagus-behandlung. Arch Ohr-Nas-u Kehlk-Heilk. 1953;163:140.
22. Dohlman G, Mattsson L. The endoscopic operation for hypopharyngeal diverticula. A roent-gencinematographic study. Arch Otolaryngol Head Neck Surg. 1960;71:744–52.
23. Weerda H, Pedersen P, Wehmer H, Braune H. A new laryngoscope for endolaryngeal micro-surgery. A contribution to injector respiration (author's transl). Arch Otorhinolaryngol. 1979;225:103–677.
24. Collard JM, Otte JB, Kestens PJ. Endoscopic stapling technique of esophagodiverticulostomy for Zenker's diverticulum. Ann Thorac Surg. 1993;56:573–6.
25. Martin-Hirsch DP, Newbegin CJ. Autosuture GIA gun: a new application in the treatment of hypopharyngeal diverticula. J Laryngol Otol. 1993;107:723–5.
26. Scher RL, Richtsmeier WJ. Endoscopic staple-assisted esophagodiverticulostomy for Zenker's diverticulum. Laryngoscope. 1996;106:951–6.
27. Mulder CJ, den Hartog G, Robijn RJ, Thies JE. Flexible endoscopic treatment of Zenker's diverticulum: a new approach. Endoscopy. 1995;27:438–42.
28. Ishioka S, Sakai P, Maluf-Filho F, Melo JM. Endoscopic incision of Zenker's diverticula. Endoscopy. 1995;27:433–7.
29. Ishak S, Hassan C, Antonello A, et al. Flexible endoscopic incision for Zenker's diverticulum: a systematic review and meta-analysis. Gastrointest Endosc. 2016;83:1076–89.
30. Costamagna G, Iacopini F, Bizzotto A, et al. Prognostic variables for the clinical success of flex-ible endoscopic septotomy of Zenker's diverticulum. Gastrointest Endosc. 2016;83:765–73.

Anatomy, Embryology, and Pathophysiology

2

Hayley Born and Rebecca J. Howell

Anatomy, Embryology, and Pathophysiology

Diverticula of the hypopharynx, most commonly Zenker diverticula (ZD), are a relatively rare disorder of the upper alimentary tract. There is an annual incidence of 2 per 100,000 patients diagnosed with ZD and much less frequent incidence of other hypopharyngeal diverticula, such as Killian-Jamieson (KJ) or Laimer's diverticula (LD) [1–3].

The named cervical diverticula can be defined by location. Each diverticulum occurs at an area of weakness in the pharyngeal or esophageal wall (Fig. 2.1). ZD occur in the area called Killian's triangle, a potential space found between the inferior pharyngeal constrictor muscle and the cricopharyngeus muscle (CPM), which together with the intrinsic musculature of the upper esophagus form the high-pressure pharyngoesophageal segment of the alimentary tract, also known as the upper esophageal sphincter (UES) [4]. The UES is a 2- to 5-cm-long region that is tonically contracted at rest and relaxed during deglutition both due to inhibition of tonic contracture of the CPM and movement of the larynx and cricoid cartilage superiorly. The inferior constrictor muscle extends from the oblique line of the thyroid cartilage to the midline pharyngeal raphe. The cricopharyngeus does not attach to a raphe, instead forms a sling attached to either side of the cricoid cartilage. For this reason, it is believed to contribute to the formation of ZD in the Killian's dehiscence above the sling, but below the raphe (Fig. 2.2). The sac of a ZD extends posterior to the cervical esophagus at or near the midline and extends into the retropharyngeal space [5–13]. The ZD usually lies just off midline, typically on the left side, although an association with handedness has been suggested [14]. The male predominance of ZD (about 1.5–3:1 male/female) [15, 16] and perhaps even the higher prevalence in places where the overall population is taller (Northern Europe, United States, Canada,

H. Born · R. J. Howell (✉)
Department of Otolaryngology, University of Cincinnati, Cincinnati, OH, USA
e-mail: Hayley.born@uc.edu; Rebecca.howell@uc.edu

© Springer International Publishing AG, part of Springer Nature 2018
R. Scher, D. Myssiorek (eds.), *Management of Zenker and Hypopharyngeal Diverticula*, https://doi.org/10.1007/978-3-319-92156-3_2

Fig. 2.1 Posterior
hypopharyngeal and
esophageal anatomy
revealing the regions of
weakness formed by the
inferior constrictor,
cricopharyngeal muscle,
and the extrinsic
esophageal muscles

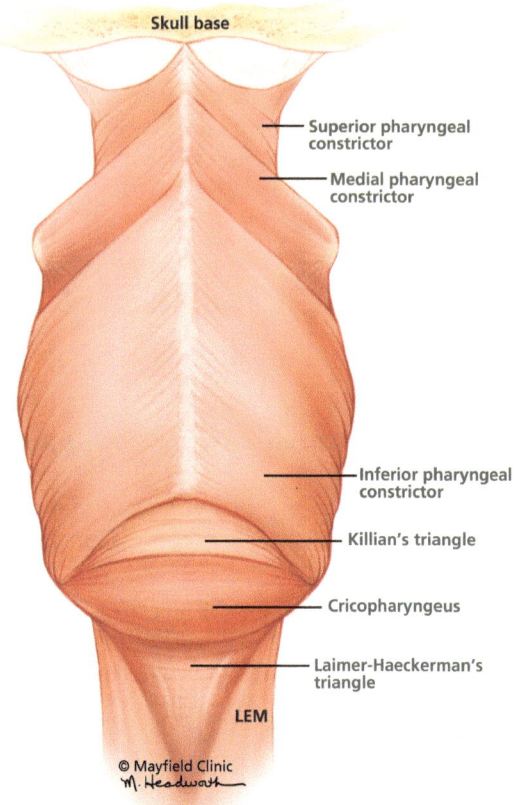

and Australia vs. Japan and Indonesia) [17] have been proposed as resulting from the difference in anthropomorphic prevalence of Killian's dehiscence [13]. The neck of the diverticular opening projects posteriorly [18].

Killian-Jamieson (KJ) diverticula, or lateral diverticula, occur in the KJ area on the anterolateral wall of the proximal esophagus inferior to the CPM, lateral to the intrinsic longitudinal muscle where it inserts onto the cricoid cartilage, and are seen lateral to the cervical esophagus (Fig. 2.2). The neck of these diverticula projects laterally from the esophagus rather than posteriorly like ZD [5, 18–20]. Lastly, LD are located in the weakened area posterior and inferior to the CPM [5]. This area, Laimer-Haeckerman's triangle, is where the posterior esophageal wall is thin, and only a single layer of circular intrinsic muscle fibers exists [20, 21]. Diverticula in this area are rare.

Hypopharyngeal diverticula can also be categorized by histology. A true diverticula involves all three layers of the esophagus, whereas a false diverticulum consists of only the mucosa and submucosa. The histology of the ZD shows the stratified squamous epithelial mucosa and the submucosa and occasionally some fibrous

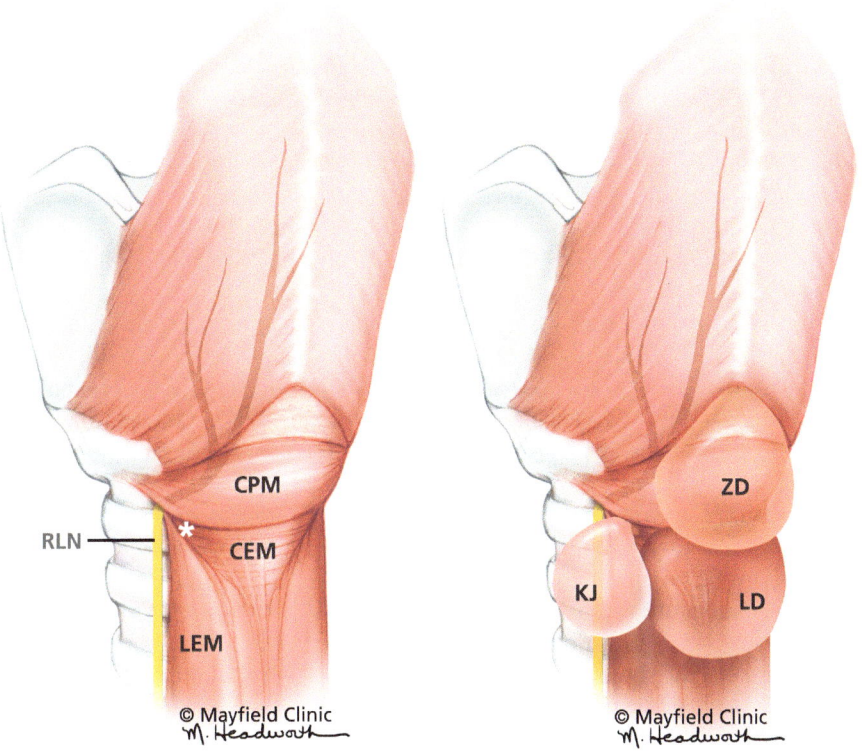

Fig. 2.2 Oblique view of the hypopharynx and esophagus (*RLN* recurrent laryngeal nerve, *CPM* cricopharyngeal muscle, *CEM* circular esophageal muscle, *LEM* longitudinal esophageal muscle, *KJ* Killian-Jamieson diverticulum, *LD* Laimer diverticulum, *ZD* Zenker diverticulum; *asterisk* area of weakness through which Killian-Jamieson diverticula exit (printed with permission from Mayfield Clinic)

tissue. The occasional muscle fiber may be present near the neck of the pouch. It is therefore classified as a false diverticulum. A KJ diverticulum, on the other hand, was originally described by Ekberg and Nylander as a true diverticulum with muscular elements [20]. Other series have described these outpouchings as projecting between sets of muscle fibers and therefore are classified as false diverticulum [12]. Management is not dependent on histological diverticulum type.

Diverticula of the hypopharyngeal area are also categorized by proposed pathophysiology, either pulsion, caused by increased intraluminal pressure or traction caused by external tension on the esophagus. Traction diverticula are rare in the hypopharynx and are only seen as secondary to other pathologic processes (e.g., trauma or malignancy) and will not be discussed in detail here. ZD is described and widely accepted to be a pulsion diverticulum, and KJ and LD are thought to be the same, though this has been questioned due their position distal to the CPM [5]. The pathophysiology of these rarer hypopharyngeal diverticula is not well understood.

The details of the pathogenesis of ZD have been widely examined in the literature. It is accepted that these are the result of high intrabolus pressure in the hypopharynx [22]. Theories regarding CPM discoordination, hyperfunction, or contraction, contributions of hereditary conditions, and association with reflux and distal strictures of the esophagus and gastroesophageal junction have been discussed. However no clear consensus has been made as to the underlying cause of the increased intraluminal pressure [23]. There is even a proposed genetic or hereditary component to ZD formation [15, 24, 25]. It is likely that ZD are the result of a combination of factors.

It is clear that the cricopharyngeal muscle plays a large role in the formation of the pulsion ZD as the point of restriction in the hypopharynx. This muscle, along with the striated muscle which forms the muscularis propria of the upper esophagus and UES, is formed from the mesenchymal layer of the fourth, fifth, and sixth branchial arches. Predictably, then, the UES innervation comes from the vagus nerve, fifth branchial arch nerve, and the recurrent laryngeal nerve (RLN), sixth branchial arch nerve [26]. This explains the correlation of swallowing dysfunction to injury of the RLN after, for example, cardiac or thyroid surgery [27]. The normal innervation occurs as follows.

As mentioned previously, the CPM is tonically contracted. During a normal swallow, a food bolus is detected by the glossopharyngeal and vagal afferent fibers in the oropharynx. In the dorsal medulla, the nerves synapse in the nucleus tractus solitarius, and interneurons carry signal to the vagal motor nuclei. Efferent signaling along neurons causes an inhibitory signal in the striated muscle fibers of the CPM just prior to the food bolus arriving. It relaxes as the strap muscles contract to cause the larynx to elevate and move anteriorly, further opening the area of the CPM. The UES dilates and opens upon passage of the bolus followed by the descent of the larynx and closure of the CPM to its tonically contracted state [7]. Disruption in any part of this reflex arc, mechanical or neurologic, are could cause increased pressure to build up in the hypopharynx anterior to Killian's triangle [28]. Normal aging or an accumulation of neurologic insults in the elderly can also disrupt this process and may contribute to the higher incidence of ZD with age [9, 29].

Incoordination of this swallow mechanism due to inadequate relaxation of the UES in swallowing has been proposed as an etiology for formation of ZD. Studies of coordination abnormalities, usually described as premature or incomplete relaxation of the UES, have also been problematic and of variable quality [29–34]. There have been several manometric studies examining the pressures in the UES during swallow in ZD patients with inconsistent results. UES pressure was found not to be correlated with ZD formation compared to patients without ZD when all these studies were considered as a group [30]. A videofluoromanometric study did show that intrabolus pressure was increased and UES opening reduced in ZD patients [35]. Overall, however, manometry has not been proven to be a useful tool in evaluating ZD or its orgins. Other techniques to measure the degree of UES dysfunction have been used such as the pharyngeal constriction ratio (PCR). PCR is calculated using fluoroscopic imaging. The ratio is derived by measuring the "pharyngeal area (including residual bolus material) visible in the lateral radiographic view at the point of maximum pharyngeal constriction during swallow (PAmax) divided by the area with a 1-cm^3 bolus held in the oral cavity (PAhold)." [36] It has been proposed as an alternate outcome measure of ZD, and the normalization of this ratio is thought to be a good surrogate for successful treatment outcome [37].

Intrinsic abnormalities of the CPM have been noted in ZD patients. In a normal person, the CPM is a striated muscle consisting predominantly of slow tonic type 1 fibers and prominant fibroadipose tissue with elastic fibers [38, 39]. In ZD patients, biopsies of the CPM have shown increased fibrosis [40, 41]. Some of these changes may be a result of gastroesophageal reflux (GER). Additionally, other biochemical changes are seen in patients with CPM disorders and UES dysfunction. Venturi et al. described an increased ratio of isodesmosine and collagen to elastin in CPM fibers [42]. They predicted that this suggests possible pathologic changes to CPM which might result in ZD.

GER has been proposed as a contributor to ZD formation. Conflicting studies exist regarding the effect of GER on CPM pressures [43, 44]. Additionally, no rigorous data regarding esophageal pH in patients with ZD has been obtained. There does, however, seem to be a higher incidence of GER in ZD patients when compared to the general population, 22–95% vs. 7% [45–49]. The criteria for diagnosing GER in these patients were not consistent. Despite this, all studies found a significantly higher prevalence of GER in ZD patients than in the general population. It is important to note that both conditions could have a related underlying cause and that correlation does not equal causation. On the other hand, several studies have directly shown that esophageal acid exposure can cause increases in UES pressure, though the underlying mechanism remains unknown [43, 50, 51]. It may be due to CPM spasm.

As described above, the pathogenesis of ZD and other hypopharyngeal diverticuli is not well understood. While there is no clear consensus of the pathogenesis of this condition, prevailing theories were described above. More than likely, a variety of factors contribute to its formation. Generally speaking, a weakened area in the muscular hypopharyngeal wall and an increase in intraluminal pressures are the only universally accepted factors in the pathogenesis of these anomalies.

Summary

This chapter focuses on the anatomy, embryology, and pathophysiology associated with hypopharyngeal diverticula. Details of the anatomy of the muscular wall of the hypopharynx, the embryologic origins of these structures, and how these relate to the intraluminal processes of swallowing are important in understanding the theories of development of hypopharyngeal diverticuli. The histology of the normal and abnormal tissues have been examined as well as manometric data relating to normal and abnormal patients. While no consensus exists for why and how hypopharyngeal diverticuli form, examining the embryology, histology, and basic anatomy can lead to an understanding of prevailing theories.

References

1. Achem SR, DeVault KR. Dysphagia in aging. J Clin Gastroenterol. 2005;39:357–71.
2. Bloom JD, Bleier BS, Mirza N, et al. Factors predicting endoscopic exposure of Zenker's diverticulum. Ann Otol Rhinol Laryngol. 2010;119:736–41.
3. Watemberg S, Landau O, Avrahami R. Zenker's diverticulum: reappraisal. Am J Gastroenterol. 1996;91:1494–8.
4. Belafsky PC, Rees CJ, Allen J, et al. Pharyngeal dilation in cricopharyngeus muscle dysfunction and Zenker diverticulum. Laryngoscope. 2010;120:889–94.
5. Undavia S, Anand SM, Jacobson AS. Killian-Jamieson diverticulum. Laryngoscope. 2013;123:414–7.
6. Dantas RO, Cook IJ, Dodds WJ, et al. Biomechanics of cricopharyngeal bars. Gastroenterology. 1990;99:1269–74.
7. Kahrilas PJ. Upper esophageal sphincter function during antegrade and retrograde transit. Am J Med. 1997;103:56S–60S.
8. Lang IM, Shaker R. Anatomy and physiology of the upper esophageal sphincter. Am J Med. 1997;103:50S–5S.
9. Plant RL. Anatomy and physiology of swallowing in adults and geriatrics. Otolaryngol Clin North Am. 1998;31:477–88.
10. Sasaki CT. Understanding the motor innervation of the human cricopharyngeus muscle. Am J Med. 2000;108:38–9.
11. Sivarao D, Goyal RK. Functional anatomy and physiology of the upper esophageal sphincter. Am J Med. 2000;108:27–37.
12. Rubesin SE, Levine MS. Killian-Jamieson diverticula: radiographic findings in 16 patients. Am J Roentgenol. 2001;177:85–9.
13. Anagiotos A, Preuss SF, Koebke J. Morphometric and anthropometric analysis of Killian's triangle. Laryngoscope. 2010;120:1082–8.
14. Stafford ND, Moore-Gillon V, McKelvie P. Handedness and the side on which pharyngeal pouches occur. Br Med J (Clin Res Ed). 1984;288:815–6.
15. van Overbeek JJ. Pathogenesis and methods of treatment of Zenker's diverticulum. Ann Otol Rhinol Laryngol. 2003;112:583–93.
16. Haidar YM, Handwerker J, Verma S. A patient with cough and dysphagia. JAMA Otolaryngol Head Neck Surg. 2014;140:673–4.
17. Verhaegen VJ, Feuth T, van den Hoogen FJ, et al. Endoscopic carbon dioxide laser diverticulostomy versus endoscopic staple-assisted diverticulostomy to treat Zenker's diverticulum. Head Neck. 2011;33:154–9.
18. Rodgers PJ, Armstrong WB, Dana E. Killian-Jamieson diverticulum: a case report and a review of the literature. Ann Otol Rhinol Laryngol. 2000;109:1087–91.
19. Udare AS, Mondel PK, Badhe PV. Killian-Jamieson diverticulum. Indian J Gastroenterol. 2014;33:98.
20. Ekberg O, Nylander G. Lateral diverticula from the pharyngo-esophageal junction area. Radiology. 1983;146:117–22.
21. Kumoi K, Ohtsuki N, Teramoto Y. Pharyngo-esophageal diverticulum arising from Laimer's triangle. Eur Arch Otorhinolaryngol. 2001;258:184–7.
22. Stewart K, Sen P. Pharyngeal pouch management: an historical review. J Laryngol Otol. 2016;1(30):116–20.
23. Schindler A, Mozzanica F, Alfonsi E, et al. Upper esophageal sphincter dysfunction: diverticula–globus pharyngeus. Ann N Y Acad Sci. 2013;1300:250–60.
24. Klockars T, Sihvo E, Mäkitie A. Familial Zenker's diverticulum. Acta Otolaryngol. 2008;128:1034–6.
25. Björk H. Pathogenesis of hypopharyngeal diverticulum with special reference to heredity. Acta Otolaryngol. 1952;42:202–7.
26. Kuo B, Urma D. Esophagus-anatomy and development. GI Motility online. 2006. https://www.nature.com/gimo/contents/pt1/full/gimo6.html

27. Hammond CS, Davenport PW, Hutchison A, Otto RL. Motor innervation of the cricopharyngeus muscle by the recurrent laryngeal nerve. J Appl Physiol. 1997;83:89–94.
28. Veenker EA, Andersen PE, Cohen JI. Cricopharyngeal spasm and Zenker's diverticulum. Head Neck. 2003;25:681–94.
29. Walters DN, Battle JW, Portera CA, Blizzard JD, Browder IW. Zenker's diverticulum in the elderly: a neurologic etiology? Am Surg. 1998;64:909–11.
30. Fulp S, Castell D. Manometric aspects of Zenker's diverticulum. Hepatogastroenterology. 1992;39:123–6.
31. Jackson C, Shallow TA. Diverticula of the oesophagus, pulsion, traction, malignant and congenital. Ann Surg. 1926;83:1–19.
32. Lund WS. The cricopharyngeal sphincter: its relationship to the relief of pharyngeal paralysis and the surgical treatment of the early pharyngeal pouch. J Laryngol Otol. 1968;82:353–67.
33. Asherson N. Achalasia of the cricopharyngeal sphincter: a record of cases, with profile pharyngograms. J Laryngol Otol. 1950;64:747–58.
34. Belsey R. Functional disease of the esophagus. J Thorac Cardiovasc Surg. 1966;52:164–88.
35. Cook IJ, Gabb M, Panagopoulos V, Jamieson GG, Dodds WJ, Dent J, Shearman DJ. Pharyngeal (Zenker's) diverticulum is a disorder of upper esophageal sphincter opening. Gastroenterology. 1992;103:1229–35.
36. Leonard R, Rees CJ, Belafsky P, et al. Fluoroscopic surrogate for pharyngeal strength: the pharyngeal constriction ratio (PCR). Dysphagia. 2011;26:13–7.
37. Venkatesan NN, Evangelista LM, Kuhn MA, Belafsky PC. Normal fluoroscopic appearance status post-successful endoscopic Zenker diverticulotomy. Laryngoscope. 2017;127:1762–6.
38. Brownlow H, Whitmore I, Willan P. A quantitative study of the histochemical and morphometric characteristics of the human cricopharyngeus muscle. J Anat. 1989;166:67–75.
39. Kristmundsdottir F, Mahon M, Froes M, Cumming WJ. Histomorphometric and histopathological study of the human cricopharyngeus muscle: in health and in motor neuron disease. Neuropathol Appl Neurobiol. 1990;16:461–75.
40. Cook I, Blumbergs P, Cash K, Jamieson GG, Shearman DJ. Structural abnormalities of the cricopharyngeus muscle in patients with pharyngeal (Zenker's) diverticulum. J Gastroenterol Hepatol. 1992;7:556–62.
41. Zaninotto G, Costantini M, Boccu C, Anselmino M, Parenti A, Guidolin D, Ancona E. Functional and morphological study of the cricopharyngeal muscle in patients with Zenker's diverticulum. Br J Surg. 1996;83:1263–7.
42. Venturi M, Bonavina L, Colombo L, et al. Biochemical markers of upper esophageal sphincter compliance in patients with Zenker's diverticulum. J Surg Res. 1997;70:46–8.
43. Gerhardt DC, Shuck TJ, Bordeaux RA, et al. Human upper esophageal sphincter. Gastroenterology. 1978;75:268–74.
44. Stanciu C, Bennett JR. Upper oesophageal sphincter yield pressure in normal subjects and in patients with gastro-oesophageal reflux. Thorax. 1974;29:459–62.
45. Ellis FH, Gibb FP, Williamson WA. Current status of cricopharyngeal myotomy for cervical eSsophageal dysphagia. Eur J Cardiothorac Surg. 1996;10:1033–9.
46. Migliore M, Payne H, Jeyasingham K. Pathophysiologic basis for operation on Zenker's diverticulum. Ann Thorac Surg. 1994;57:1616–20.
47. Lerut T, Van Raemdonck D, Guelinckx P, et al. Zenker's diverticulum: Is a myotomy of the cricopharyngeus useful? How long should it be? Hepatogastroenterology. 1992;39:127–31.
48. Williams RB, Ali GN, Hunt DR, et al. Cricopharyngeal myotomy does not increase the risk of esophagopharyngeal acid regurgitation. Am J Gastroenterol. 1999;94:3448–54.
49. Resouly A, Braat J, Jackson A, et al. Pharyngeal pouch: link with reflux and oesophageal dysmotility. Clin Otolaryngol Allied Sci. 1994;19:241–2.
50. Wallin L, Boesby S, Madsen T. The effect of HCl infusion in the lower part of the oesophagus on the pharyngo-oesophageal sphincter pressure in normal subjects. Scand J Gastroenterol. 1978;13:821–6.
51. Willing J, Davidson G, Dent J, Cook I. Effect of gastro-oesophageal reflux on upper oesophageal sphincter motility in children. Gut. 1993;34:904–10.

Diagnosis and Evaluation of Hypopharyngeal Diverticula

3

David Myssiorek and Laurie Wennerholm

Introduction

Hypopharyngeal diverticula are uncommon. Their incidence has been estimated to be 2/100,000 in the United States [1]. They tend to be more prevalent in men with a male to female estimated ratio of 1.5–1 [2]. There appears to be a different incidence geographically as well. Northern Europeans are more prone to Zenker diverticula (ZD) than southern Europeans. Compared to the United States, Canada, and Australia, the incidence is much lower in Japan and Indonesia [3]. While the most common presentation is during the seventh to eighth decades, ZD have been found throughout adulthood. Perhaps there may be genetic contributions as there have been reports of hypopharyngeal diverticula occurring in families [4, 5].

As covered elsewhere in this book, there are two types of diverticula of the hypopharynx: pulsion and traction. Traction diverticula were associated with tuberculosis and retropharyngeal adenopathy in the past but more recently have been most commonly associated with anterior surgical approaches for cervical spine disease [6]. Adhesion of the posterior pharynx to the cervical spine hardware can lead to development of a diverticulum. In extreme cases, the hardware and screws can be found within the traction sac (Fig. 3.1). Since they are traction diverticula, they are represented by all three layers of the posterior wall of the hypopharynx. While less common, they must be suspected during the evaluation of any hypopharyngeal diverticulum.

D. Myssiorek (✉)
Jacobi Medical Center, Bronx, NY, USA

Department of Otolaryngology, Albert Einstein College of Medicine, Bronx, NY, USA

L. Wennerholm
Speech Pathology and Swallowing Center for Cancer Care, White Plains Hospital/Montefiore Health System, White Plains, NY, USA
e-mail: Lwennerhol@wphospital.org

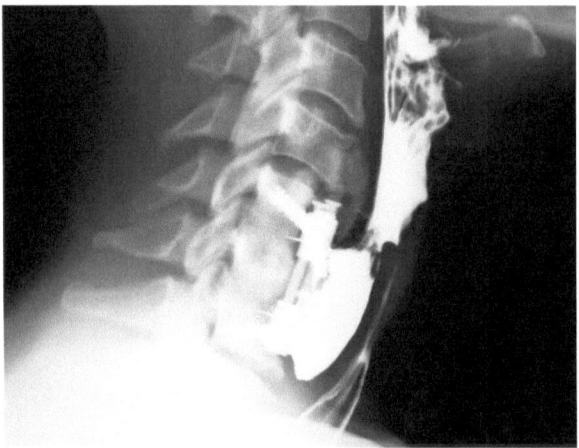

Fig. 3.1 Traction diverticulum secondary to surgery for cervical spine injury

History

All hypopharyngeal diverticula present similarly. The patient most commonly presents with dysphagia. Some patients may be referred for an incidental finding of a diverticulum found during a flexible esophagoscopy performed for other causes. Computed tomographic imaging for unassociated pathology may detect a diverticulum. In obtaining a history, the patient's age, sex, and heredity may raise the suspicion of a hypopharyngeal diverticulum.

Regurgitation of undigested food is the sine qua non for Zenker diverticulum. Gurgling is a prominent complaint and can sometimes be heard while the patient sleeps. Other symptoms include weight loss, excessive throat mucus and throat clearing, coughing, and halitosis. Symptoms may be of recent onset or be present for years. A history of previous cervical surgery or transmural infections of the esophagus is easily obtained. Prior surgery of the thyroid and parathyroid glands, carotid arterial system or larynx should be sought. These will impact potential open approaches to a diverticulum. Currently it is unclear if gastro-esophageal reflux is causal with regard to hypopharyngeal diverticula, but patients should be questioned about this possibility as it could certainly impact posttreatment symptom relief.

Physical Examination

A routine physical examination of the head and neck should be performed. Attention to dentition, jaw excursion, and any other obstructions in the oral cavity or oropharynx needs to be recorded. Loose or broken teeth require addressing especially when considering endoscopic treatment of ZD. If the patient is to undergo transoral treatment of their diverticulum, some dentists can create a custom-fitting dental guard. The benefit of this device is that it can be used to protect the upper teeth from excessive force from the endoscope. It will usually have a lower profile than the dental guards available in most operating theaters.

Reduced jaw excursions may make transoral treatment difficult to impossible. Certain patients with stocky necks do not have jaw excursion wide enough to admit a rigid laryngoscope but may admit a flexible scope. Therefore, examination of the jaw and neck is essential to determining operability of some patients. Neck range of motion requires examination. Severely kyphotic patients will not permit placement of rigid endoscopes for transoral treatment (Fig. 3.2). This condition is not correctable with anesthetic relaxation.

Visualization of the hypopharynx should be performed but rarely adds to the diagnosis. However, vocal fold mobility is assessed which is particularly important if an open procedure is entertained. Frequently, mucus pooling in the hypopharynx is visualized. This may clear with swallowing, but then quickly reappears due to collection in the diverticulum. Rarely, the orifice of the diverticulum can be visualized in an office setting, especially with non-Zenker diverticula, since the diverticular opening is inferior to the cricopharyngeal muscle.

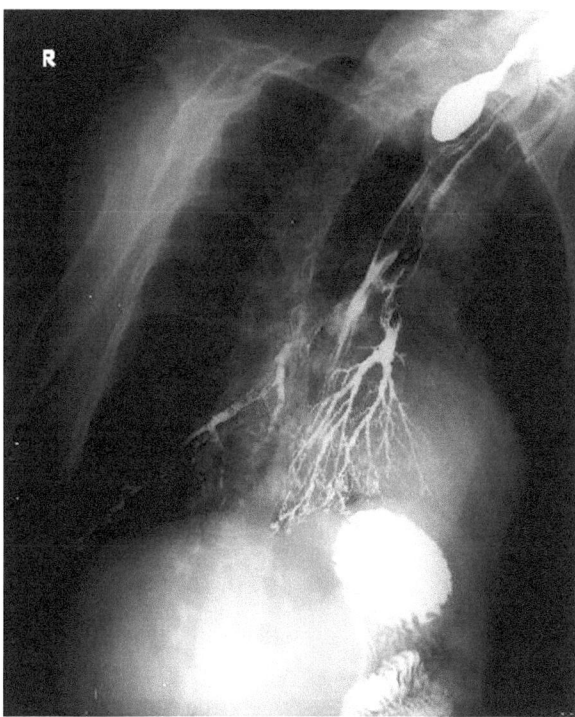

Fig. 3.2 Kyphotic patient with a Zenker diverticulum

Diagnosis

Radiologic Imaging

Establishment of the diagnosis of a hypopharyngeal diverticulum is confirmed with radiologic imaging. The gold standard is a barium esophagram with cine-esophagography (Fig. 3.3). Some patients aspirate during these studies (Fig. 3.4). For this reason, barium is preferred over water-soluble agents such as gastrografin. Gastrografin is caustic to lung tissue and should be avoided. The diverticulum is identified, its size is determined, and the size of the diverticular opening is assessed. It is critical to determine the position of the diverticulum in the event that an open

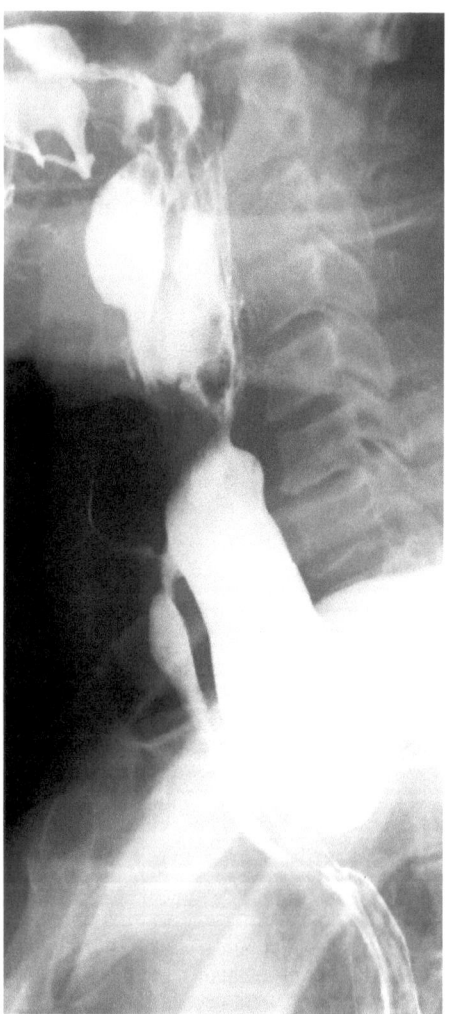

Fig. 3.3 Esophagram of large Zenker diverticulum, sagittal or lateral view

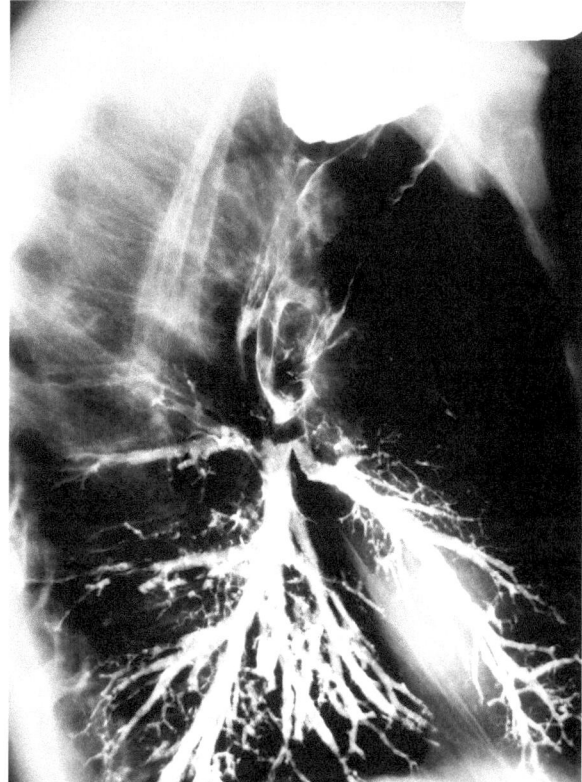

Fig. 3.4 Esophagram revealing aspiration of contrast

procedure is elected. Approximately 10% of ZD present on the right side (Fig. 3.5). More importantly, the relationship of the cricopharyngeal muscle relative to the neck of the diverticulum is essential. If the cricopharyngeal muscle is above the neck of the diverticulum, then it is not a ZD (Fig. 3.6a, b). A diverticulum that localizes below the cricopharyngeal muscle should be examined in the AP and lateral projection. In the AP projection, the diverticulum may be seen lateral to the esophagus which would be consistent with a Killian-Jamieson diverticulum. If it is imaged well in the lateral projection, and below the cricopharyngeal muscle, it is a rare Laimer diverticulum. This obviously would impact treatment and is covered elsewhere in this book.

A classic ZD will be found at the midline, at the pharyngoesophageal junction (Fig. 3.7). The classic view is the lateral view which will demonstrate the sac at approximately the level of the fifth and sixth cervical vertebrae. Cine-esophagography will reveal a narrow esophagus immediately anterior to and below the opening of the ZD. As the diverticula expand, they lateralize to the left approximately 90% of the time. Uncommonly, a large diverticulum will sequester the entire bolus of barium preventing evaluation of the esophagus unless more

Fig. 3.5 Esophagram, AP
view of a Zenker
diverticulum presenting on
the right side

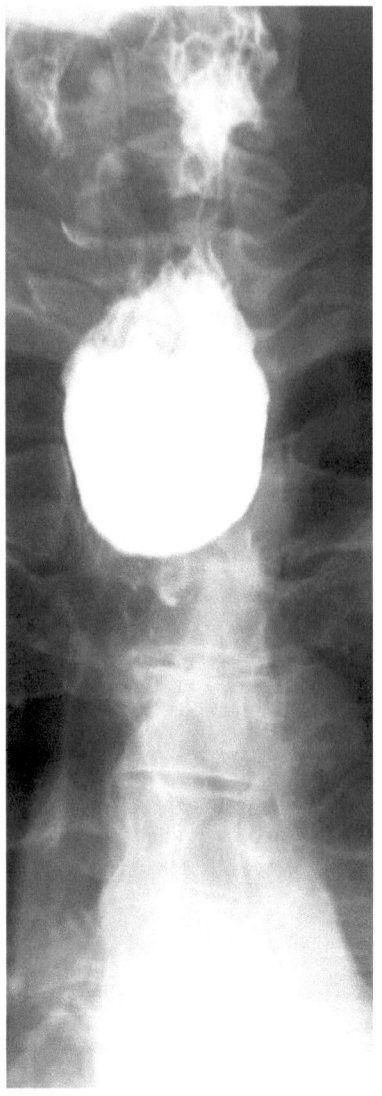

barium is delivered. Smaller diverticula may not be imaged adequately if they are superimposed on the esophageal barium bolus. An experienced radiologist will rotate the patient slightly to an oblique plane to better visualize small diverticula. Although rare, cancers found in ZD can present as an irregularity of the sac lumen on the lateral projection. Most institutions perform videofluoroscopy making review of the study easier. Downstream observation of the study may show other intrinsic abnormalities of the esophagus including dysmotility and distal strictures.

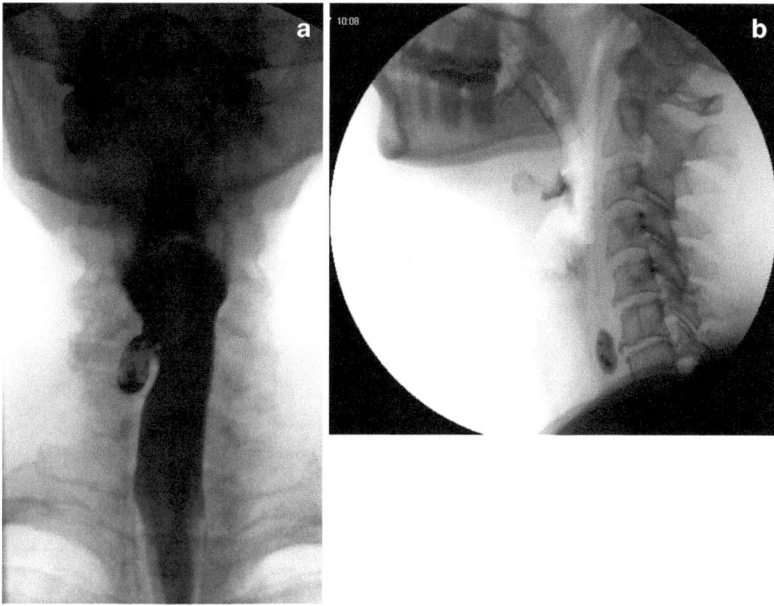

Fig. 3.6 (a) Reverse barium esophagram of a Killian-Jamieson diverticulum presenting laterally. (b) Sagittal view of same patient

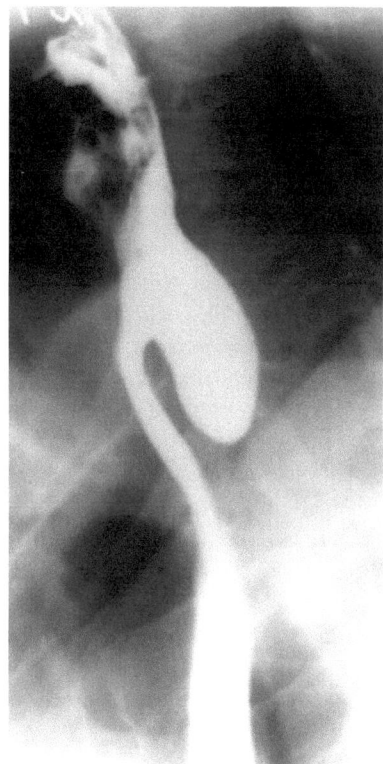

Fig. 3.7 Esophagram of a classic Zenker diverticulum

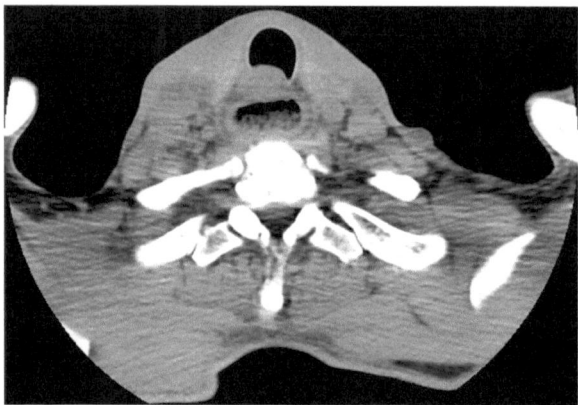

Fig. 3.8 Computed tomogram of a Zenker diverticulum filled with gas and debris. The esophagus is outlined between the diverticulum and the posterior trachea

Computed tomographic scanning (CT) is not usually used for diagnosis of ZD but may be useful for KJD. Asymptomatic patients being imaged for other entities of the thorax and neck may incidentally identify a ZD. The diverticulum will contain particulate matter and gas. It localizes between the spine and the esophagus (Fig. 3.8). Since the trachea and larynx are anterior to the esophagus, the esophagus can be visualized between two air-filled cavities. This air contrast can show a thickened upper esophagus indenting the trachea and suggesting the thickness of the upper esophageal sphincter. If there is evidence of cancer in the sac, CT scanning will help delineate local involvement and adenopathy.

Ultrasound has been used to detect ZD, although it is not currently recommended for routine clinical assessment. Ultrasound contrast agent is ingested by the patient, and the patient is scanned. At this time, oral use of SonoVue (Bracco, Milan, Italy) is off label. As expected, the diverticulum appears posterior to the hypopharynx and esophagus and retains contrast for greater than 3 min [7]. The procedure can be performed without the need for a radiology suite, and the patient is not exposed to radiation. However, the study does not offer the detail of a barium study and cannot visualize the position of a diverticulum relative to the cricopharyngeal muscle. The images are not as easily interpreted during operative treatment of hypopharyngeal diverticula.

Scintigraphy of ZD has been employed. Scintigraphy has been used to evaluate esophageal motility issues. Valenza et al. compared scintigraphic identification of ZD to barium studies [8]. Technetium-99m colloid was swallowed as a bolus, and the patient was imaged. Ninety-four percent of the patients studied were correctly identified. The authors claimed that the study was less costly, exposed the patient to less radiation, and was better tolerated by elderly patients than either barium studies or manometry. However, the images offer less detail and are difficult to interpret with regard to the other hypopharyngeal diverticula.

The authors highly recommend bringing the images of the barium radiographic study to the operating theater in all cases of operative management. Sidedness of the sac and the size of the diverticular orifice compared to the esophageal inlet are critical when endoscopically approaching these diverticula for treatment.

Manometry

Esophageal manometry is an important tool in evaluating esophageal motility. It does have limited application in evaluating hypopharyngeal diverticula [9]. In a study by Broll et al., after myotomy and sac excision of ZD, preoperative manometric pressure was decreased [10]. Ishioka et al. studied five patients with ZD evaluated manometrically before and after endoscopic treatment [11]. The mean pressure of the upper esophageal sphincter preoperatively was 54.6 cm water with a length of 3 cm. Post-diverticulotomy, that pressure decreased to 26.8 cm of water [12]. In another study, following transoral treatment of ZD, 30 patients had a significant drop in mean resting pressure of the cricopharyngeal muscle [13]. From a starting pressure of 16.23 mmHg, on average it fell to 9.26 mmHg. The intrabolus pressure at the cricopharyngeal muscle decreased from 22.48 to 10.16 mmHg.

While these studies add to our knowledge of the pathophysiology of ZD and our ability to predict outcomes, they do not add to the diagnostic evaluation of hypopharyngeal diverticula. Therefore, they are not currently recommended in the evaluation of these diverticula.

Diverticula and the Speech-Language Pathologist

In the 1980s the speech-language pathologist (SLP) became one of the main professionals responsible for the evaluation and treatment of dysphagia, specifically oropharyngeal dysphagia [14]. Since then, for decades, the SLP has worked in conjunction with the otolaryngologist and gastroenterologist to determine the nature and location of the swallowing deficit.

The two most common methods for the SLP to use to visualize the swallow are the modified barium swallow study (MBSS) and the fiber-optic endoscopic evaluation of swallow (FEES). The MBSS was created by Jeri Logemann and her colleagues by "flipping up" the image of an esophagram to view the oropharyngeal swallow and the cervical esophagus [12]. The test is performed in real time and differs from the barium swallow in that it is not a series of still images.

The FEES was created by Susan Langmore [14] to improve portability of formal swallowing evaluations using a flexible laryngoscope to view the endolarynx and its surrounding tissues. The SLP endoscopist views the path of the bolus and patterns of residue, while the patient is swallowing green- or blue-dyed food stuffs. Together with the patients' symptoms, imaging like the MBS and FEES reveals a variety of oral, pharyngeal, and esophageal phase disorders. There are specific findings on each exam that aid in the diagnosis of the ZD, such as residual bolus in the vallecula signalling deficits in tongue base to posterior pharyngeal wall contact.

Early symptomatology may be vague and nonspecific, "Something sticks in my throat." This is consistent with a symptom that accompanies many pharyngeal or esophageal issues from reflux to pharyngeal and esophageal dysfunction. A cricopharyngeal bar may obstruct flow of pills during swallowing and may be a sign of an early ZD. As the pouch becomes larger, the patient may complain that food sticks in the throat and it may be regurgitated (especially if the patient bends at the waist) [15]. In addition, the patient may complain of dysgeusia, an intermittent bad taste in the mouth as well as halitosis.

MBSS or videofluoroscopic evaluation of the swallow can provide extremely useful information about the size and impact of a ZD on swallowing physiology [16, 17]. On MBSS, in the lateral plane, the oropharyngeal swallow may be intact, with a bolus collection that forms a barium-filled pouch in the region of the hypopharynx/cricopharyngeus. Depending upon the size of the pouch and depth, the pouch may empty after the swallow and then fill again during the next swallow. In fact, according to Sydow et al., most material that accumulates will exit upward through the defect's inlet and reenter the hypopharynx eliciting a secondary swallow [18]. If the pouch becomes filled to capacity, it will be partially or completely aspirated after the swallow.

ZD are not common reasons for most patients' dysphagia. With prevalence between 0.01 and 0.11%, less experienced SLPs may not connect the clinical signs and reported symptoms with imaging findings to reveal the defect. One reason is the inferior location of the pouch. The laryngopharynx contracts and raises two to three vertebral levels of height during the swallow and then falls within 1–2 s [19]. Since the ZD is at the level or below the CP, the pouch may not be easily viewed. Placing a patient in a lateral oblique view to eliminate shoulder obstruction can significantly improve the view and reveal the ZD [15].

Another hallmark sign that a ZD may be present on an MBSS is a pattern of post swallow "refilling" of the distal pharynx in the absence of retention in the proximal pharynx. For example, a patient who has delayed post-swallow leakage of material from the valleculae to the pyriform sinuses may have reduced tongue base retraction and clearance of the valleculae on swallow offset. However, the patient with a ZD would have no such pattern of top to bottom spillage. According to Coyle, the SLP may focus too closely on the airway and miss aspiration originating from an inferior and lateral source, that being a ZD [15]. One final sign of a possible ZD on videofluoroscopic swallow evaluation is post-swallow aspiration that does not have a clear origin.

Vaezi indicated that endoscopy will not contribute to diagnosis of diverticulum and may place a patient at risk for perforation of the pouch [16]. In addition, Perie and colleagues noted that direct viewing of the diverticulum is difficult on endoscopy in that the structures are collapsed upon each other at rest and in swallowing [20]. The pouch may reside lower than the endoscope allows. However, in their study, a group of 12 patients demonstrated a manifestation of a ZD on endoscopy that aided in differential diagnosis. Patients were seen for FEES and viewed while ingesting a cream bolus. Authors described the "sign of the rising tide" as a manifestation of a ZD during which the bolus completely clears the pharynx and several seconds later reappears. Authors confirmed the diagnosis via the standard fluoroscopic study. Of note, this was found to be a specific sign for ZD, and it was not present after surgical diverticulectomy.

Unlike oral and pharyngeal phase swallowing disorders that result from stroke or head and neck cancer, muscular strengthening exercises may not be appropriate in cases of diverticula, and they oftentimes require surgical intervention. However, consistency modification, postures, and maneuvers that can be outlined by an SLP as well as counseling can reduce a patient's aspiration risk and improve feeding quality [15, 21]. In their study, Holmes and colleagues found that SLPs were able to reduce risk of aspiration in patients with diverticula using liquid or solid modification and swallowing strategies. Coyle outlined the use of head rotation and increased bolus volume as behavioral techniques to improve clearance of the ZD, thereby reducing the residual in the pouch and the risk of large-volume aspiration. Typically, in head rotation, the patient is cued to turn the head to the damaged hemipharynx to divert the bolus down the stronger hemipharynx [22]. Another outcome of head rotation as determined by manometry is that it lowers the resting pressure of the UES and delays UES closing. In head rotation, the patient benefits from reduced resistance to bolus flow from the upper sphincter as well as a lengthier duration of esophageal opening [23]. These combined effects can enhance pharyngoesophageal clearance and aid in the behavioral emptying of a ZD. There are occasions when the patient may actually benefit from a head rotation to the stronger side. Coyle suggests trialing head rotation in both directions to assess benefit. Improvement would be determined by the height of the post-swallow residue within the pouch as compared to the pouch height. The higher the contrast level, the greater the risk for post-swallow aspiration. In addition to postural changes like head rotation and airway protection strategies, cued or deliberate cough and re-swallow can assist in providing greater clearance of a penetrant or aspirant. In practice, improving a patient's understanding of his/her need to cough and re-swallow can improve safety if this strategy is integrated into feeding tasks. Therefore, in select cases, behavioral interventions can be used in the treatment of ZD. This is particularly important if the patient is not appropriate for surgery. In these cases, the role of the SLP in the management of a patient with ZD becomes magnified, and he/she must have the tools to optimize function via traditional, behavioral techniques that, when used in combination, may have an impact on health status of the patient and his/her quality of life.

References

1. Achem SR, DeVault KR. Dysphagia in aging. J Clin Gastroenterol. 2005;39:357–71.
2. Klockars T, Sihvo E, Mäkitie A. Familial Zenker's diverticulum. Acta Otolaryngol. 2008;128:1034–6.
3. van Overbeek JJ. Pathogenesis and methods of treatment of Zenker's diverticulum. Ann Otol Rhinol Laryngol. 2003;112:583–93.
4. Feussner H, Siewert JR. Zenker's diverticulum and reflux. Hepatogastroenterology. 1992;39:100–4.
5. Björk H. Pathogenesis of hypopharyngeal diverticulum with special reference to heredity. Acta Otolaryngol. 1952;42:202–7.
6. Alexander RE, Silber J, Myssiorek D. Staged surgical management of hypopharyngeal traction diverticulum. Ann Otol Rhinol Laryngol. 2008;117:731–3.

7. Cui X, Ignee A, Baum U, Dietrich CF. Feasibility and usefulness of using swallow contrast-enhanced ultrasound to diagnose Zenker's diverticulum: preliminary results. Ultrasound Med Biol. 2015;41:975–81.

8. Valenza V, Perotti G, Di Guida D, Castrucci G, Celi G, Restaino G. Scintigraphic evaluation of Zenker's diverticulum. Eur J Nucl Med Mol Imaging. 2003;30:1657–64.

9. Fulp SR, Castell DO. Manometric aspects of Zenker's diverticulum. Hepatogastroenterology. 1992;39:123–6.

10. Broll R, Kramer T, Kalb K, Bruch HP. Manometric follow-up after resection of Zenker's diverticulum. Z Gastroenterol. 1992;30:142–6.

11. Ishioka S, Felix VN, Sakai P, Melo J, Pinotti HW. Manometric study of the upper esophageal sphincter before and after endoscopic management of Zenker's diverticulum. Hepatogastroenterology. 1995;42:628–32.

12. Logemann J. Evaluation and treatment of swallowing disorders. 2nd ed. Austin: Pro-Ed; 1998.

13. Ozgursoy OB, Salassa JR. Functional and manofluorographic outcomes after transoral endoscopic pharyngoesophageal diverticulostomy. Arch Otolaryngol Head Neck Surg. 2010;136:463–7.

14. Langmore S. Endoscopic evaluation and treatment of swallowing disorders. 1st ed. New York: Theime; 2001.

15. Coyle J. Zenker's diverticulum. In: Jones H, Rosenbek J, editors. Dysphagia in rare conditions: an encyclopedia. San Diego: Plural Publishing; 2010. p. 671–80.

16. Vaezi M. Esophageal Diseases: an atlas of investigation and management. Oxford: Clinical Publishing; 2006.

17. Cook IJ. Cricopharyngeal function and dysfunction. Dysphagia. 1993;8:244–51.

18. Sydow BD, Levine MS, Rubesin SE, Laufer I. Radiographic findings and complications after surgical or endoscopic repair of Zenker's diverticulum in 16 patients. AJR. Am J Roentgenol. 2001;177:1067–71.

19. Leonard R, Kendall K, McKenzie S. UES opening and cricopharyngeal bar in nondysphagic elderly and nonelderly adults. Dysphagia. 2004;19:182–91.

20. Perie S, Dernis HP, Angelard B. The "sign of the rising tide" during swallowing fiberoscopy: a specific manifestation of Zenker's diverticulum. Ann Otol Rhinol Laryngol. 1999;108:296–9.

21. Holmes E, Kenny C, Samuel M, Regan J, O'Rourke J, McCoubrey C. The role of speech and language therapy in assessing and managing pharyngo-esophageal diverticula. Ir Med J. 2015;108:296–9.

22. Logemann J, Kahrilas BR, Kobara M, Vakil N. The benefit of head rotation on pharyngo-esophageal dysphagia. Arch Phys Med Rehabil. 1989;70:767–71.

23. Ohmae Y, Ogura M, Kitahara S. Effects of head rotation on pharyngeal function during the normal swallow. Ann Otol Rhinol Laryngol. 1998;107:344–8.

Treatment of Cricopharyngeal Muscle Dysfunction

Tawfiq Khoury, C. Scott Brown, and Seth M. Cohen

Introduction

The role of the cricopharyngeal (CP) muscle in swallowing has been known since 1717 when Valsalva fist described the anatomy and function of the CP muscle [1]. Killian in 1907 then further clarified the anatomy and function of the CP muscle and laid the groundwork for what we know today. CP muscle dysfunction is attributable to an abnormal tightening of the cricopharyngeus which makes up the majority of the upper esophageal sphincter (UES) [2, 3]. This can lead to dysphagia, weight loss, and even aspiration which in turn can be a source of significant morbidity and can lead to a drastic reduction in quality of life [4]. There are three events that need to occur in order for the UES to open: First is a neurologic phase in which there is neural inhibition of the intrinsically contracted sphincter [2, 3]. Then, the extra-laryngeal musculature functions to move the larynx anteriorly and superiorly serving to mechanically open the inlet of the UES. Finally, a bolus passes and passively stretches the UES. The etiology of cricopharyngeal dysfunction is widely variable, and anything that disrupts any of the three steps mentioned above can lead to decreased UES function [5]. Neurologic entities such as stroke, parkinsonism, diabetic neuropathy, myasthenia gravis, and many others can impact tonic relaxation and laryngeal elevation. Other patients suffer from a neoplastic process which may invade vital nerves or mechanically block the UES leading to dysfunction. Individuals who have undergone radiation to the neck can have fibrosis or denervation of the cricopharyngeal musculature which leads to CP dysfunction. Other individuals may have evidence of the condition with no discernable underlying cause.

T. Khoury · C. S. Brown · S. M. Cohen (✉)
Division of Head and Neck Surgery and Communication Sciences, Department of Surgery, Duke University Medical Center, Durham, NC, USA
e-mail: seth.cohen@duke.edu

© Springer International Publishing AG, part of Springer Nature 2018
R. Scher, D. Myssiorek (eds.), *Management of Zenker and Hypopharyngeal Diverticula*, https://doi.org/10.1007/978-3-319-92156-3_4

Presentation

A variety of preoperative techniques can be used to evaluate a patient for CP dysfunction, and while there is debate in the literature as to what a full evaluation should entail, it is widely accepted that the most important part of the workup is the history [6–11]. Patients frequently present with dysphagia for solids, liquids, or both [5]. Weight loss can be seen in many patients. Clinical evaluation will typically include a full head and neck examination as well as a flexible laryngoscopy. These exams may show pooled secretions in the pyriform sinuses or postcricoid region and may identify signs of an underlying neurological condition or neoplasms. In the absence of a specific underlying cause on history and physical examination, it is common to have the patients undergo a videofluoroscopic swallowing study (VFSS) which can not only demonstrate UES dysfunction but can also be used to evaluate laryngeal elevation, pharyngeal muscle strength, and signs of aspiration or laryngeal penetration (Fig. 4.1). The utility of high-resolution manometry is debated in the literature. McKenna et al. noted clinical and fluoroscopic data was sufficient to make the diagnosis and treat patients [6]. Other authors including Olsson et al. have demonstrated that the position of the manometry probe is crucial to obtaining accurate results and pressure can vary widely with even small changes in probe positioning [7]. Salassa et al. proposed a set of standards for manometric equipment and fluoroscopic guidance to help alleviate this variability and improve the utility of manometry in the diagnosis of CP dysfunction [12]. In general, we feel that manometry should be used in borderline cases where there is not a clear-cut diagnosis based on history, physical examination, and fluoroscopy. In these instances, demonstration of increased CP pressure on manometry can help determine if a patient is a candidate for procedural intervention. In addition, good pharyngeal strength may portend a good outcome [13]. Patients with suspected underlying neurological disorders may in some cases benefit from electromyography of the cricopharyngeus and inferior constrictor during swallowing, but though this practice may be helpful in some select cases, it is not widely used [14, 15]. Other adjuncts such as CT scans or laboratory evaluations are not generally performed unless there is suspicion for an underlying neoplastic, rheumatologic, or otherwise systemic disease contributing to the patient's cricopharyngeal dysfunction.

Treatment Overview

There are several options available to patients with cricopharyngeal dysfunction. These include use of botulinum toxin injection, CP dilation, endoscopic CP myotomy, and open CP myotomy. Botulinum toxin has been employed with good effect [4]. This technique first gained popularity after being reported by Schneider in 1994 [16]. The effective duration and the dosage of toxin used vary, but most studies use between 5 and 100 units of botulinum A toxin injected into the CP muscle [3, 17, 18]. Many studies have reported good outcomes, and, though several systematic reviews have shown that other procedures have a higher success rate, this remains a good option for many patients [5]. Botox may be a suitable option for

Fig. 4.1 Radiographic appearance demonstrating impression from the cricopharyngeus (CP)

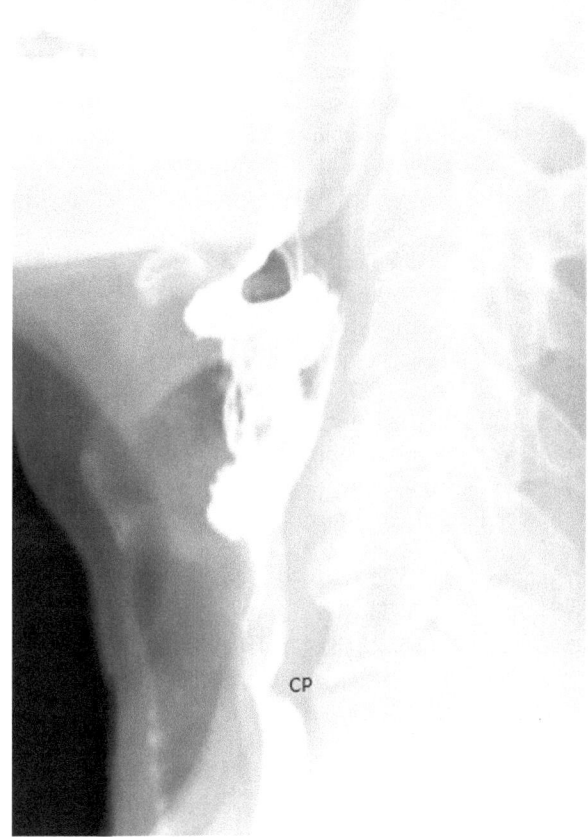

patients who do not want more invasive myotomy or as a possible intermediate step to determine the impact of addressing CP hypertonicity on overall swallowing function prior to a myotomy.

Another treatment option for patients includes either balloon or rigid dilation of the UES. This has the advantage of being able to be performed under light sedation as opposed to general anesthesia and has a lower complication rate than either endoscopic or open CP myotomy [13]. Though there are few studies comparing this method to the others, Wang et al. found that in his cohort when a patient had CP dysfunction attributable only to a CP bar on fluoroscopy, dilation provided a complete response [19]. Dilation can also be combined with botulinum toxin injection.

Despite the newer treatments available, the treatment with the highest success rate remains CP myotomy [5, 20, 21]. In a systematic review, Kocdor et al. noted that myotomy had a higher success rate at 75% than either Botox (69%) or dilation (73%), though only the difference with respect to myotomy and Botox was statistically significant. Furthermore, the authors noted that endoscopic myotomy had a higher success rate than open myotomy. Though the procedures seem to be the most effective based on the current literature, a patient's specific situation must be taken into account before recommending any intervention.

Endoscopic Trans-Oral Approaches

The endoscopic approach to the CP muscle dates back to 1917 when it was first described by Mosher for treatment of Zenker's diverticulum (ZD) [22]. Mosher abandoned this procedure after his seventh patient died of mediastinitis. In 1951, Kaplan was credited with performing the first CP myotomy for the treatment of CP dysfunction using a similar method [23]. CP myotomy techniques continued to improve for the treatment of both CP dysfunction and ZD. Dohlman and Mattson readopted and popularized the procedure in 1960 when they published 100 patients treated for ZD without complications [24]. Suture-less endoscopic approaches did not gain popularity at that time due to fear of mediastinitis. Several refinements in technique have been applied to endoscopic CP myotomy which reduce these concerns [16, 24–27]. Dohlman and Mattson, for example, used diathermic coagulation to divide the CP muscle. Many advances have been made since that time: van Overbeek et al. used a CO_2 laser to divide the CP muscle in 1984, while Bent and Kuhn described using a KTP laser for the same purpose in 1992 [28, 29].

Several different trans-oral endoscopic techniques have been described for the definitive treatment of CP dysfunction. Despite variations in technique and equipment, the goal of all of these approaches is generally the same—divide the CP muscle. The patient is positioned in the supine position, and general endotracheal anesthesia is induced. The bed is typically turned 90° counterclockwise for a right-handed surgeon with anesthesia positioned to the left of the patient and the instrument table to the patient's right. A shoulder roll may be placed for neck extension. Standard laser safety precautions are used for cases employing laser division. We typically use the Weerda laryngoscope, which is the precursor to modern endoscopic diverticuloscopes and is slightly shorter than most of the available diverticuloscopes. The Weerda laryngoscope is otherwise operated the same and has two adjustment screws that control distal and proximal scope apertures. The screw on the backside functions to cantilever the blades of the laryngoscope and is used to open the distal end. The screw on the side pushes the blades apart and is used to open the entire length of the scope. The scope is placed in the post cricoid area and opened until a view of the esophagus and cricopharyngeus muscle is obtained (Fig. 4.2). The laryngoscope is then suspended on a mustard table or a Mayo stand. At this point several options exist to divide the CP muscle. We typically use a carbon dioxide (CO_2) laser set at 4 W continuous, but other settings are also frequently used [30]. The pulsed mode of the laser improves visualization at the expense of speed. Electrocautery, steel, and potassium titanyl phosphate (KTP) lasers have also been used for this purpose, but we find that the CO2 laser offers excellent hemostasis as well as good visualization of the plane of the cricopharyngeus muscle as it is divided. Complete division of the CP muscle is performed until the buccopharyngeal fascia is seen (Fig. 4.3). All instrumentation is then removed from the patient, and the patient is turned back to anesthesia and awakened. Flexible endoscopic techniques have also been described using the CO_2 laser, and these techniques can be particularly helpful in patients where exposure is difficult with a rigid diverticuloscope [31].

Fig. 4.2 Endoscopic view demonstrating the esophageal inlet (E) and prominent cricopharyngeus (CP)

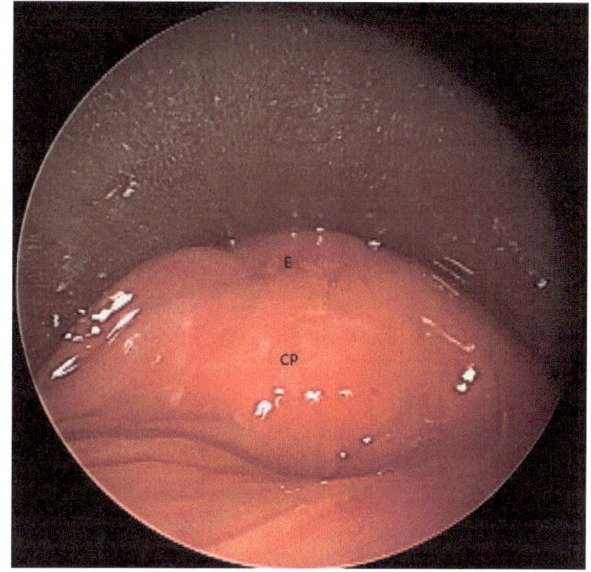

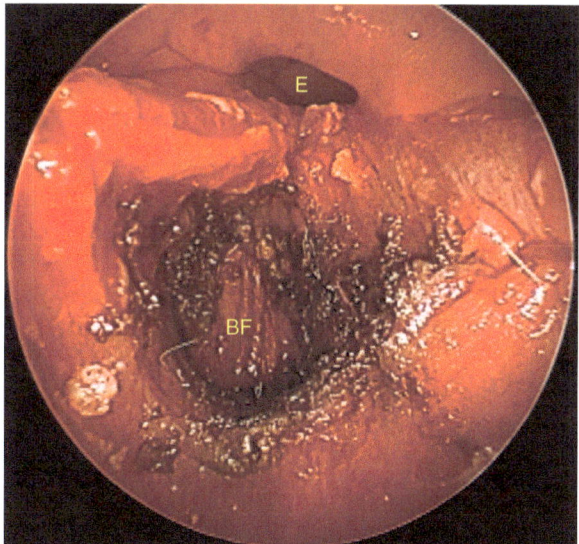

Fig. 4.3 Endoscopic view demonstrating completion of cricopharyngeal myotomy. Muscle fibers are incised to the buccopharyngeal fascia (BF). Esophageal lumen (E)

Postoperative care varies between institutions. We typically hospitalize the patient overnight and restart a liquid diet on postoperative day 1. If the patient's vital signs remain stable and the patient is otherwise feeling well on postoperative day 1, the patient is discharged on a full liquid diet with instructions to continue full liquids until follow-up at 3 weeks. Several studies have evaluated outpatient endoscopic CP myotomy and, in appropriately selected patients, have not shown any additional adverse effects [32]. The procedure has a good outcome for most patients. Hoesseini et al. did a retrospective review of 47 cases and found that 85% of patients experienced symptom relief postoperatively [33]. Twenty-five percent of patients developed recurrent symptoms requiring a second procedure. All 40 patients who experienced symptom relief postoperatively were eventually satisfied with treatment after an average of 1.3 surgeries. Complications using this technique are rare. Pitman et al. reviewed a nine-patient series and noted 12% had complications including one aspiration pneumonia, one transient vocal fold paralysis, and one mortality secondary to pneumonia [30]. Though esophageal leak and mediastinitis are potential complications, these are rare using this technique as even if the buccopharyngeal fascia is violated, there remains undisturbed retropharyngeal tissue which serves to contain leaks. This is in contrast to an open CP myotomy in which all layers are disturbed. There are also mucosal closure techniques that can be performed after the myotomy [4].

The Open Approach

Appropriate patient selection is critical for the success of treatment for CP dysfunction. Due to certain patient anatomic characteristics, such as micrognathia or the inability to extend the neck, endoscopic techniques may not be possible. Patients must be counseled that some of these factors may not be clear until they are evaluated and examined in the operating room. If an endoscopic approach cannot be safely performed, conversion to an open approach may be needed. Due to the typical older age of patients with CP dysfunction, comorbidities and other patient health factors should be considered prior to proceeding to this approach. In particular, patients with significant pulmonary problems or uncontrolled reflux may benefit from extensive respiratory therapy and anti-reflux medications before and after surgery.

In order to perform the surgery, perioperative antibiotics should be administered to minimize postoperative wound infection, especially in the event that a pharyngotomy is made. The patient should be laid supine on the operative table and a shoulder roll used to facilitate gentle extension of the neck. A rigid esophagoscopy should be performed for several reasons. First, neoplasms and other inflammatory esophageal diseases should be excluded as cause of dysphagia, even if CP achalasia has been confirmed with radiographic studies. Second, a 36 Fr Maloney dilator (Medovations, Milwaukee, WI, USA) is passed into the esophagus in order to assist with intraoperative identification and to provide additional width and tension to help with the myotomy.

Externally, the patient's thyroid and cricoid cartilages should be palpated if possible. A transverse cervical incision should then be made at the level of the cricoid cartilage. This incision should typically be offset to the patient's left side. Subplatysmal flaps are then raised to a superior limit of the thyroid notch and inferiorly to a level near or at the clavicle. The anterior border of the sternocleidomastoid (SCM) is identified and the fascia divided. Isolating the SCM from the strap muscles allows for the SCM and carotid sheath to be retracted laterally. The laryngotracheal complex can then be retracted to the opposite side, allowing visualization of the retropharyngeal space. We typically divide the superior belly of the omohyoid, reducing the tension of retraction.

The loose connective tissue is then dissected down to the level of the prevertebral fascia. Blunt dissection will facilitate exposure of the pharyngeal musculature. With the Maloney dilator in the esophagus, it can be easily palpated. The horizontal fibers of the cricopharyngeus distinguish it from the inferior constrictor, which is obliquely oriented. With the muscle exposed, a small hemostat can be used to separate a plane between the pharyngeal mucosa and the CP (Fig. 4.4). The entire length of the CP should be divided extending into the inferior constrictor and esophageal muscles in order to prevent recurrence.

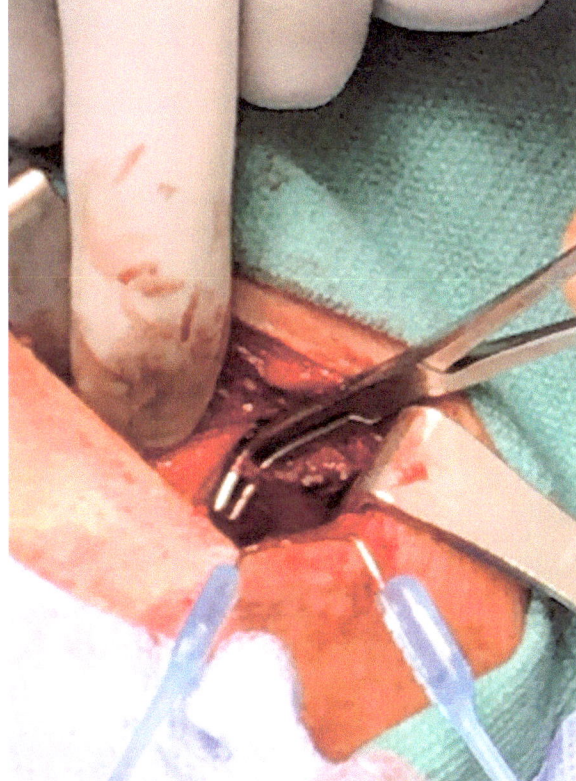

Fig. 4.4 Transcervical approach to cricopharyngeal myotomy. The cricopharyngeal muscle is exposed by the hemostat

Postoperatively, the patient is kept overnight in the hospital or discharged on the same day. On the morning of the first postoperative day, a gastrografin swallow study may be performed to ensure that there is no pharyngeal leak. The patient is then provided with a clear liquid diet and discharged after removing the drain. After 48 h of a clear liquid diet, the patient is instructed to advance to full liquids for 48 h and to a soft diet as tolerated thereafter. They are seen in follow-up 3 weeks later to reassess symptoms.

Risks of CP myotomy via the open approach include pharyngeal leakage, recurrent laryngeal nerve injury, and incomplete CP division leading to persistent or recurrent dysphagia [34]. The risk of these immediate complications is quite low, despite the generalized poor nutrition of this particular patient population. Pulmonary complications are the most common, occurring in 5–10% of patients. In an analysis of 250 patients undergoing CP myotomy, Brigand et al. noted that respiratory complications occurred only in patients with myogenic dysphagia [35]. Retropharyngeal fluid collections and inflammation, as well as fistula, may also occur, though are significantly less likely. Outcomes of success vary among published studies. Several theories for this variability have been proposed. The underlying cause of a patient's dysfunction (muscular vs. neurological) may impact their outcome. In properly selected patients, however, the success rate approaches 75% [36]. This variability reemphasizes the importance of appropriate history and patient selection for the procedure.

Summary

Cricopharyngeal muscle dysfunction can have significant negative impact on patients' swallowing function. Various options for treating cricopharyngeal muscle dysfunction include dilation alone or with botulinum toxin and myotomy which can be performed endoscopically or transcervically. As dysphagia is a complex problem, shared decision-making between the clinician and patient can determine the best course of action.

References

1. Lim KG. The mouth of the esophagus. Laryngoscope. 1907;17:421–8.
2. Munoz AA, Shapiro J, Cuddy LD, et al. Videofluoroscopic findings in dysphagic patients with cricopharyngeal dysfunction: before and after open cricopharyngeal myotomy. Ann Otol Rhinol Laryngol. 2007;116:49–56.
3. Alberty J, Oelerich M, Ludwig K, et al. Efficacy of botulinum toxin A for treatment of upper esophageal sphincter dysfunction. Laryngoscope. 2000;110:1151–6.
4. Ho AS, Morzaria S, Damrose EJ. Carbon dioxide laser-assisted endoscopic cricopharyngeal myotomy with primary mucosal closure. Ann Otol Rhinol Laryngol. 2011;120:33–9.
5. Kocdor P, Siegel ER, Tulunay-Ugur OE. Cricopharyngeal dysfunction: a systematic review comparing outcomes of dilatation, botulinum toxin injection, and myotomy. Laryngoscope. 2016;126:135–41.

6. Lim RY. Endoscopic CO2 laser cricopharyngeal myotomy. J Clin Laser Med Surg. 1995;13:241–7.
7. Olsson R, Nilsson H, Ekberg O. An experimental manometric study simulating upper esophageal sphincter narrowing. Invest Radiol. 1994;29:630–5.
8. Ozgursoy OB, Salassa JR. Manofluorographic and functional outcomes after endoscopic laser cricopharyngeal myotomy for cricopharyngeal bar. Otolaryngol Head Neck Surg. 2010;142:735–40.
9. Hatlebakk JG, Castell JA, Spiegel J, et al. Dilatation therapy for dysphagia in patients with upper esophageal sphincter dysfunction-manometric and symptomatic response. Dis Esophagus. 1998;11:254–9.
10. McKenna JA, Dedo HH. Cricopharyngeal myotomy: indications and technique. Ann Otol Rhinol Laryngol. 1992;101:216–21.
11. Kos MP, David EF, Klinkenberg-Knol EC, Mahieu HF. Long-term results of external upper esophageal sphincter myotomy for oropharyngeal dysphagia. Dysphagia. 2010;25:169–76.
12. Salassa JR, DeVault KR, McConnel FM. Proposed catheter standards for pharyngeal manofluorography (videomanometry). Dysphagia. 1998;3:105–10.
13. Ali GN, Wallace KL, Laundl TM, Hunt DR, deCarle DJ, Cook IJ. Predictors of outcome following cricopharyngeal disruption for pharyngeal dysphagia. Dysphagia. 1997;12:133–9.
14. Ertekin C, Aydogdu I, Yuceyar N, et al. Electrodiagnostic methods of neurogenic dysphagia. Electroencephalogr Clin Neurophysiol. 1998;109:331–40.
15. Poirier NC, Bonavina L, Taillefer R, et al. Cricopharyngeal myotomy for neurogenic oropharyngeal dysphagia. J Thorac Cardiovasc Surg. 1997;113:233–40.
16. Aly A, Devitt PG, Jamieson GG. Evolution of surgical treatment for pharyngeal pouch. Br J Surg. 2004;91:657–64.
17. Blitzer A, Brin MF. Use of botulinum toxin for diagnosis and management of cricopharyngeal achalasia. Otolaryngol Head Neck Surg. 1997;116:328–30.
18. Haapaniemi JJ, Laurikainen EA, Pulkkinen J, Marttila RJ. Botulinum toxin in the treatment of cricopharyngeal dysphagia. Dysphagia. 2001;16:171–5.
19. Wang AY, Kadkade R, Kahrilas PJ, Hirano I. Effectiveness of esophageal dilation for symptomatic cricopharyngeal bar. Gastrointest Endosc. 2005;61:148–52.
20. Takes RP, Hoogen FJA, Marres HAM. Endoscopic myotomy of the cricopharyngeal muscle with CO2 laser surgery. Head Neck. 2005;27:703–9.
21. Lawson G, Remacle M. Ins and outs of myotomy of the upper esophageal sphincter in swallowing disorders. B-ENT. 2008;10:83–9.
22. Mosher HP. Webs and pouches of the esophagus: their diagnosis and treatment. Surg Gynecol Obstet. 1917;25:175–87.
23. Kaplan S. Paralysis of deglutition, a post-poliomyelitis complication treated by section of the cricopharyngeus muscle. Ann Surg. 1951;133:572.
24. Dohlman G, Mattson O. The endoscopic operation for hypopharyngeal diverticula. Arch Otolaryngol Head Surg. 1960;71:744–52.
25. Morton RP, Bartley JRF. Inversion of Zenker's diverticulum: the preferred option. Head Neck. 1993;15:253–6.
26. Payne S, Reynolds R. Surgical treatment of pharyngoesophageal diverticulum [Zenkers diverticulum]. Surg Rounds. 1982;5:18–24.
27. Negus VE. Pharyngeal diverticula. Observations on their evolution and treatment. Br J Surg. 1950;38:129–46.
28. Overbeek v, Jos JM, Hoeksema PE, Edens ET. Microendoscopic surgery of the hypopharyngeal diverticulum using electrocoagulation or carbon dioxide laser. Ann Otol Rhinol Laryngol. 1984;93:34–6.
29. Kuhn FA, Bent JP. Zenker's diverticulotomy using the KTP/532 laser. Laryngoscope. 1992;102:946–50.
30. Pitman M, Weissbrod P. Endoscopic CO2 laser cricopharyngeal myotomy. Laryngoscope. 2009;119:45–53.

31. Juzgado Lucas D. Flexible endoscopic cricopharyngeal myotomy - The gold standard for the management of Zenker's diverticulum. Rev Esp Enferm Dig. 2016;108:295–6.
32. Gross ND, Cohen JI, Andersen PE. Outpatient endoscopic Zenker diverticulotomy. Laryngoscope. 2004;114:208–11.
33. Hoesseini A, Honings J, Taus-Mohamedradja R, van den Hoogen FJ, Marres HA, van den Broek GB, Kalf H, Takes RP. Outcomes of endoscopic cricopharyngeal myotomy with CO2 laser surgery: a retrospective study of 47 patients. Head Neck. 2016;38:1022–7.
34. Campbell BH, Touminen TC, Toohill RJ. The risk and complications of aspiration following cricopharyngeal myotomy. Am J Med. 1997;103(5A):61S–3S.
35. Brigand C, Ferraro P, Martin J, Duranceau A. Risk factors in patients undergoing cricopharyngeal myotomy. Br J Surg. 2007;94:978–83.
36. Bhattacharyya N. Cricopharyngeal myotomy treatment & management. https://emedicine.medscape.com/article/836966-treatment#d15. Accessed 2 Jan 2018.

Open Surgery for Zenker Diverticulum

5

Molly Naunheim, Albert L. Merati, and Philip A. Weissbrod

Background

Patients with Zenker diverticulum have long been known to benefit from surgical repair, yet early attempts at transcervical treatment had significant morbidity [1]. Innovations in endoscopic surgery, such as use of the endoscopic stapler first reported in 1993 [2], allowed for transoral diverticulotomy which effectively reduced the previously high rates of complications following open surgery. Yet, as surgical sterility, device technology, and overall technique has have improved, open and endoscopic procedures have a more comparable risk profile [3]. It is an often-debated topic without clarity as to which technique is superior.

To date, there has been no randomized control trial completed to directly answer this question. Most of the data regarding surgical repair of ZD is in the form of retrospective review, often with limited follow-up. While it is easy to bemoan the lack of prospective comparative data, many have admirably examined this topic within the limitations of their clinical practice, and there is certainly much to be gleaned from these reports.

Verdonck and Morton [4] completed a systematic review in 2015 of the comparative and cohort studies on ZD treatment. Seventy-one studies were included, looking both at outcomes between groups (i.e., open vs. endoscopic) and within

M. Naunheim
Department of Otolaryngology—Head and Neck Surgery,
University of California—San Francisco, San Francisco, CA, USA

A. L. Merati (✉)
Department of Otolaryngology—Head and Neck Surgery, University of Washington School of Medicine, Seattle, WA, USA
e-mail: amerati@uw.edu

P. A. Weissbrod
Division of Otolaryngology—Head and Neck Surgery, Department of Surgery, University of California San Diego, La Jolla, CA, USA

© Springer International Publishing AG, part of Springer Nature 2018
R. Scher, D. Myssiorek (eds.), *Management of Zenker and Hypopharyngeal Diverticula*, https://doi.org/10.1007/978-3-319-92156-3_5

groups (i.e., laser vs. stapler in endoscopic repair). Rate of failure, defined as inability to manage the pouch and resolve the dysphagia, was significantly higher with endoscopic compared to open techniques, most notably in short-term failures (14.5% vs. 1.3%, respectively). Overall rates of failure were reported at 18.4% for endoscopic procedures and 4.2% for open procedures, with a minimum mean follow-up time of 12 months. Complications were more frequent in the open approach (11% vs. 7%). Types of complications were different as well, with emphysema and mediastinitis being more common following endoscopic repair and nerve palsy, fistula, and hematoma more common following open repair. Of note, this paper examined several different methods of endoscopic repair (laser, coagulation, flexible, and stapler); the risk of mediastinitis was noted to be 0.2% for stapler repair (2 of 1089 patients), 0.4% for flexible repair (1 of 251 patients), 1.5% for laser procedures (13 of 894 patients), and 3% (13 of 437 patients) when the pouch was removed with argon laser; this led to an overall risk of 1.2% during endoscopic procedures (compared to 0.3% in open procedures). The average risk of mediastinitis for endoscopic procedures was increased in this study due to inclusion of argon laser procedures. Surgery-related death rates were very low in both groups (0.9% open and 0.4% endoscopic). Length of stay was significantly shorter for those treated by endoscopic repair. This particular publication reviewed series that spanned several decades of treatments, and thus may not adequately reflect improvements in technique, changes in method preference, or current rates of complications.

Yuan et al. [5] also completed a systematic review of the literature. They identified 93 studies, totaling 6915 patients between the years of 1990 and 2011, which met their search criteria. Nineteen of these studies compared results of open and endoscopic approaches. Complications were reported in 8.7% and 10.5% of cases, respectively; mortality was reported in 0.2% of open cases and 0.6% of endoscopic cases. Reports of recurrence were not uniformly defined, and thus no conclusions were made.

Albers et al. [6] completed a meta-analysis including 11 studies, totaling 596 patients, comparing endoscopic and open techniques from 1975 to 2014. The authors concluded that endoscopic treatments required less time in the operating room, less time without a diet, and fewer complications than the open surgical treatments. Open surgical treatments, on the other hand, were associated with less recurrence. A few things should be noted about this meta-analysis. First, the majority of the 11 studies analyzed did not report means or standard deviations, and thus were not included in calculations of length of operating room procedure or time to diet. Complications were reported in all 11 studies, and only data from 1 study was removed due to heterogeneity; these complications were reported in 7.6% of endoscopic and 15.8% of open procedures. Specifically, the most common complications when assessing both approaches were cervical leak, hoarseness, aspiration pneumonia, chest pain, and esophageal perforation. All 11 studies were included in the report of recurrence; patients with ZD treated endoscopically recurred at a rate of 13%, whereas those treated with the open method had a rate of 6.4% recurrence. Mean follow-up time was not quantified. This analysis spanned greater than three decades of research studies, allowing for incorporation of many studies, yet also including shifts in practice which have accompanied endoscopic innovations.

Smaller studies have corroborated some of these findings. Chang et al. [7] examined 52 patients treated consecutively, with 28 open procedures and 24 endoscopic cases. Again, the endoscopic procedure was shorter than the open procedure (47 min compared to 170 min). No recurrences were seen for patients treated with the open procedure, but 3 of 24 patients (12.5%) treated endoscopically required revision. In this particular study, there was no difference in length of hospital stay or rate of complication. The authors concluded there is a higher likelihood of recurrence following endoscopic repair. Multiple other studies have supported this conclusion, with recurrence rates reported anywhere from 12 to 32% [8–10] for endoscopic case series. Follow-up is inconsistent between studies, however, making a direct comparison between these numbers is inadvisable.

Quality of life outcomes following the two treatments have also been investigated. Seth and colleagues in 2014 [11] surveyed postoperative patients using the gastrointestinal quality of life scale, specifically inquiring about regurgitation, halitosis, dysphagia, and choking; patients retrospectively recalled their symptoms at both 1 month postoperatively and at the time of the current follow-up phone call. Fifty-five patients with at least 1 year of follow-up were successfully contacted; mean follow-up was 5.1 years for patients who underwent open repair and 3.7 years for those who underwent endoscopic repair. All patients reported marked improvement in symptoms compared to their preoperative state, but complete resolution was reported more often by those treated with open repair (93.5% vs. 66.7%). Interestingly, those treated with endoscopic repair on average reported worsened symptoms at their follow-up phone call compared to 1 month postoperatively. The authors posited that this recurrence of symptoms is due to incomplete myotomy which may occur during the endoscopic repair; notably, all endoscopic repairs in this series were performed with the stapler. Wirth et al. [3] found similar results in their questionnaire administered to 47 patients, with dysphagia symptoms reported to be absent in 91% of open surgical patients compared to 83% of those treated with endoscopic surgery.

Voice and swallowing outcomes have also been examined between the open approach and the endoscopic approach using a laser for diverticulotomy and myotomy. Schoeff et al. [12] obtained survey data using the Voice Handicap Index 10 (VHI-10) and the Eating Assessment Tool-10 (EAT-10) both pre- and postoperatively for patients with ZD. This was a retrospective review, and only 11 patients had data sufficient for analysis. Interestingly, however, both swallowing and voice outcomes improved following surgery. The authors attribute this improved subjective quality of voice to the elderly age of most ZD patients; they suggest that subclinical, age-related dysphonia is not perceived until after surgical repair confers a slight benefit to the clarity and loudness of the patients' voice. This may be related to the often reported "wet" voice of patients with ZD, due to pooling of secretions which may overflow into the laryngeal vestibule.

While again there is no direct comparison between endoscopic and open repair of ZD, most of the current literature suggests that both approaches are relatively safe. The endoscopic repair requires a shorter operative time, and often a shorter hospital stay, but confers a greater risk of recurrence. With respect to complications, some studies show relatively equivalent complication rates [4, 5], while others suggest that the open approach has higher rates [7]. This begs the question: how should the physician and patient decide on the most appropriate treatment?

Patient factors certainly play a role in deciding which is the best approach to surgical intervention. Elderly patients or those with comorbidities have more anesthetic risk [13, 14]. In this population, endoscopic approach may be preferable due to reduced operative time and shorter hospitalization. Similarly, endoscopic procedures may be favorable in previously operated or radiated necks as the risk of complication may be increased in a scarred or radiated field. Alternatively, certain patient characteristics may favor the open approach. Anatomic factors such as poor neck extension, high body mass index (BMI), short neck, and prominent teeth may make endoscopic procedures less successful [15, 16]. Additionally, younger patients may benefit from an open approach, as recurrence rates are lower with the open approach and these patients will have many decades to develop recurrence. Therefore, each patient should be individually considered, and risks and benefits must be thoroughly discussed. Characteristics of the diverticulum also should play a role in determination of approach. Both very large and very small diverticula are likely to benefit from an open procedure. For extremely large sacs, the remnant which is left following endoscopic diverticulotomy is relatively hypotonic which creates an adynamic segment. Anecdotally, an endoscopic repair on a very large diverticulum can leave behind a poorly motile segment, though it is unclear what implication this remnant has on either function or recurrence. The authors typically encourage patients to consider open diverticulectomy for diverticula larger than 3 cm. For patients with small sacs, myotomy may be all that is necessary. Endoscopic repair in small sacs can be more challenging [5, 17–19]. While endoscopic cricopharyngeal myotomy is an option for ZD [20], van Overbeek, who performed 646 endoscopic treatments of ZD, suggested that for "patients with a small diverticulum, an external sphincterotomy (myotomy) alone is to be preferred" [21].

Indications

Dysphagia is the main indication for ZD treatment. Overtly concerning symptoms such as weight loss and aspiration pneumonia are more pressing indications for surgery, as the patient's health rather than the patient's quality of life is at risk. The aim of surgical treatment is to first improve the safety of swallow and next improve quality. Though meaningful postoperative oral intake is not always possible due to long-term outflow obstruction causing pharyngeal pump weakness, appropriate treatment can mitigate any aspiration of pooled secretions or food contents. Consideration of other swallow pathology preoperatively is relevant as esophageal dysmotility can be prominent in this population. This effectively could reduce postsurgical swallow performance, a concept that should be introduced during preoperative counseling to allow patients to have appropriate postoperative expectations.

Symptoms of dysphagia due to ZD often present in the seventh or eighth decade of life. Given the relative late presentation and likelihood of having other more pressing medical comorbidities at this age, the physician should first consider whether surgical intervention should be recommended at all. Though this is a surgical disease, unless the patient is unable to obtain adequate nutrition or is aspirating due to pharyngeal pooling, surgery is not mandatory; many patients can live long and healthy lives with their disease. If disease severity is placing patients' health at risk and surgery is recommended, the patient should then decide whether or not to pursue treatment at all based on a thorough discussion of risks and benefits. Following this, patient characteristics and diverticular size, as outlined above, should direct the discussion when deciding upon surgical approach.

Preoperative Imaging

Swallow imaging is essential for assessment of any swallow disorder. Fluoroscopic swallow evaluation allows for confirmation of presence of the diverticulum, assessment of the prominence of the cricopharyngeal muscle, estimation of the size of the diverticulum, and laterality, all important factors in the preoperative surgical decision-making process. Laterality is of particular importance for open surgery. While most ZD are left sided, there is incidence of right-side dominant lesions which can be difficult to reach via a left-sided approach. For this reason, anterior-posterior fluoroscopy is recommended in addition to the typical sagittal view.

In young, highly functioning patients, modified barium swallow (MBS) may not be necessary, and barium esophagram (BA) may suffice. In the authors' institutions, this is an easier study to obtain, reduces time of workup, and provides all necessary information. For older patients or those with more questionable swallow function, MBS or both MBS and BA may be worthwhile studies. Information regarding additional oropharyngeal or esophageal sources for dysfunction may contribute to a more informed decision-making process regarding the choice to proceed with surgery and counseling regarding postsurgical expectations of function.

Additionally, imaging can help differentiate ZD from other rarer diverticula. A Killian-Jamieson diverticulum protrudes through Killian's dehiscence *antero*laterally, under the cricopharyngeus muscle and lateral to the longitudinal tendon of the esophagus. Though symptoms may be similar when present, Killian-Jamieson pouches are more likely to be asymptomatic [22]; this may occur because the CP muscle lies above the pouch, and closure of this muscle can prevent reflux through the upper esophageal sphincter. Though the surgical approach can be somewhat similar, it is of obvious importance to distinguish whether the esophagus lies anterior or medial to the diverticulum. This diagnosis is made primarily on radiographic studies. Though this can be treated both endoscopically and open, an open approach is preferred due to the close proximity of the recurrent laryngeal nerve [23]. Pharyngocele, another hypopharyngeal diverticulum, is an outpouching in the pyriform sinus through the thyrohyoid membrane; this can present with symptoms similar to a ZD, such as dysphagia and regurgitation. Pharyngoceles are classically associated with increased luminal pressure (e.g., trumpet players) [24, 25]. Pharyngoceles, when repair is required, may also be addressed either open or endoscopically [26]. Further details of management of Killian-Jamieson diverticula and pharyngoceles are outside of the scope of this chapter.

Technique

The operation is performed in the following sequence:

1. General anesthesia is induced with the patient orotracheally intubated and the patient positioned with the head in extension.
2. Endoscopy:
    (a) Cricopharyngeal bar, sac, and esophagus are identified.
    (b) Contents inside sac are cleared.
    (c) The sac is packed with methylene blue-colored 1/4″ plain strip gauze.
    (d) A soft bougie is placed into the esophagus, 36–40 Fr, size permitting.
3. Open procedure:
    (a) A horizontal incision immediately below the level of the cricoid, approximately 4–5 cm in length, is made just left of midline extending to the anterior border of the sternocleidomastoid.
    (b) The omohyoid muscle is identified and retracted or divided.
    (c) Blunt dissection is used to create space medial to the vascular compartment and extended down to the anterior aspect of the prevertebral fascia.
    (d) The sac is then identified and completely dissected free from the pharynx and esophagus via blunt dissection.
    (e) The packing is removed transorally by a member of the operating room team.
    (f) The sac is then placed on moderate tension and removed, and the pharyngotomy is repaired (usually with a stapling device).
    (g) A full cricopharyngeal (CP) myotomy is performed with myectomy by feathering a #15 blade across the muscle until only the mucosa remains.
    (h) The bougie is removed transorally.
    (i) If desired, a feeding tube is placed trans-nasally with digital pressure placed across the anastomotic line.
    (j) The wound is irrigated and a passive drain is placed.

Detailed narrative ZD surgery is performed under general anesthesia. Use of a small endotracheal tube can improve the ease of maneuvering the endoscope. It is imperative that endoscopic evaluation be performed at the time of definitive open surgery. The hypopharynx and cervical esophagus are exposed with any one of a number of endoscopes. Two of the most useful endoscopes for visualization are the distracting Weerda diverticuloscope (Karl Storz, Tuttlingen, Germany) and the non-distracting Benjamin-Hollinger diverticuloscope (Karl Storz, Tuttlingen, Germany); both of these may be put in suspension. In cases of difficult exposure, a Miller 3 blade (an anesthesia-intubating laryngoscope) can be used to engage the cervical esophagus; this offers an excellent view of the sac and bar, but suspension is not an option. Adequate visualization of the cricopharyngeal (CP) bar can be quite difficult but is necessary for appropriate investigation of the native esophagus and sac (Fig. 5.1).

Goals of endoscopy are threefold. First, one must identify and characterize the diverticulum and position relative to the native esophagus. Next, the sac should be emptied of food contents (Fig. 5.2). Finally, other sources of obstruction should be ruled out by endoscopic inspection such as malignancy or stricture, as they can impact the decision of approach and surgical outcome (Fig. 5.3).

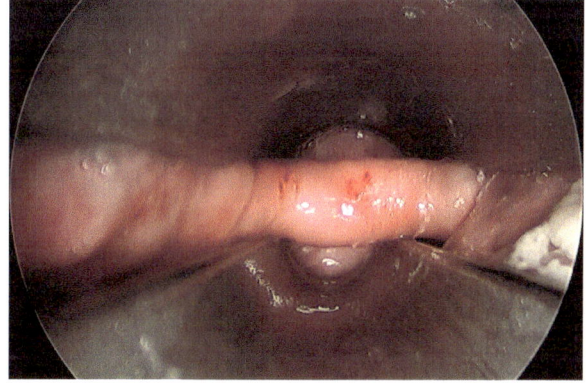

Fig. 5.1 Endoscopic view of a cricopharyngeal bar. A Weerda distending diverticuloscope is in place, putting the transverse posterior portion of the cricopharyngeal muscle—or "bar"—on tension

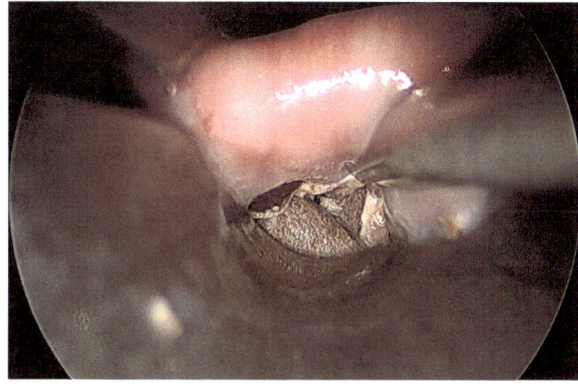

Fig. 5.2 Endoscopic view preoperatively of Zenker diverticulum with debris in the sac

Fig. 5.3 Patient with a recurrent Zenker diverticulum and esophageal stricture. following prior endoscopic approach. Jackson esophageal probe is placed anteriorly through the true esophageal lumen.

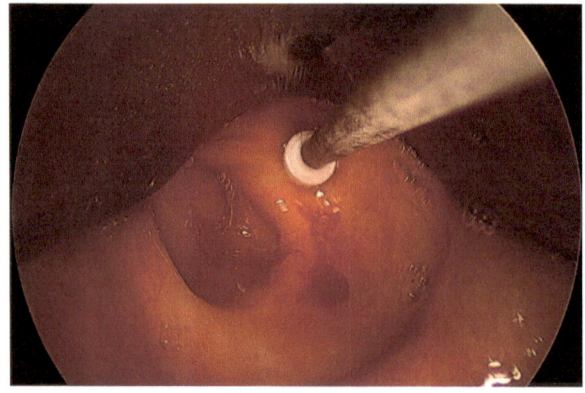

Once this is complete, the surgeon should pack the diverticulum with 1/4″ plain strip gauze colored with methylene blue-colored saline (Fig. 5.4). This packing facilitates identification and palpation during the open portion of the case. The methylene blue causes transmucosal staining of the diverticulum wall, enabling easier identification during the open surgical steps. Next, a bougie is placed in the esophagus; the authors most often use a soft Maloney dilator (36 or 38 French). One should note that the direction of the bougie may be much more anterior than anticipated because the packed diverticulum accentuates the lordosis of the cervicothoracic junction. In the rare instance where the diverticula cannot be visualized transorally, the procedure can continue with bougie placement only, however, identification of the diverticula transcervically may be difficult. When exposure of the diverticula is difficult, use of a Miller 3 can allow improved access due to its low profile as compared to more traditional laryngoscopes.

Next, the patient is prepped and draped. A 4–5 cm incision is then planned with a marking pen. A 5 cm incision is adequate for even the largest of sacs. The incision should begin a few millimeters (mm) below the cricoid on the left side of the neck and extend to the anterior border of the sternocleidomastoid muscle (SCM). The neck of the sac is at the level of the cricoid, thus an incision made directly below it affords appropriate exposure. The incision is planned on the left side of the neck for two reasons. First, the cervical esophagus gradually tracks to the left as it descends into the upper chest. Second, the course of the left recurrent laryngeal nerve (RLN) is more predictable (and possibly more stretch-resistant [27]) than the right, and there is no risk for a nonrecurrent laryngeal nerve.

Subplatysmal flaps are elevated, and the fascia is incised along the anterior border of the SCM. The omohyoid muscle is identified as it crosses the field; this should be divided if necessary for improved exposure and can be tagged for later repair. A tunnel is then created in the visceronvertebral angle using blunt dissection, similar to an anterior approach to the spine; no traction should be placed on the tracheoesophageal groove so as not to cause injury to the RLN. Throughout this maneuver, the vascular compartment should not be disturbed. Once the spine is

Fig. 5.4 (**a**) Endoscopic view of esophagus anteriorly, cricopharyngeal bar, and posterior sac. (**b**) Methylene blue-soaked plain strip gauze packed into the sac posteriorly

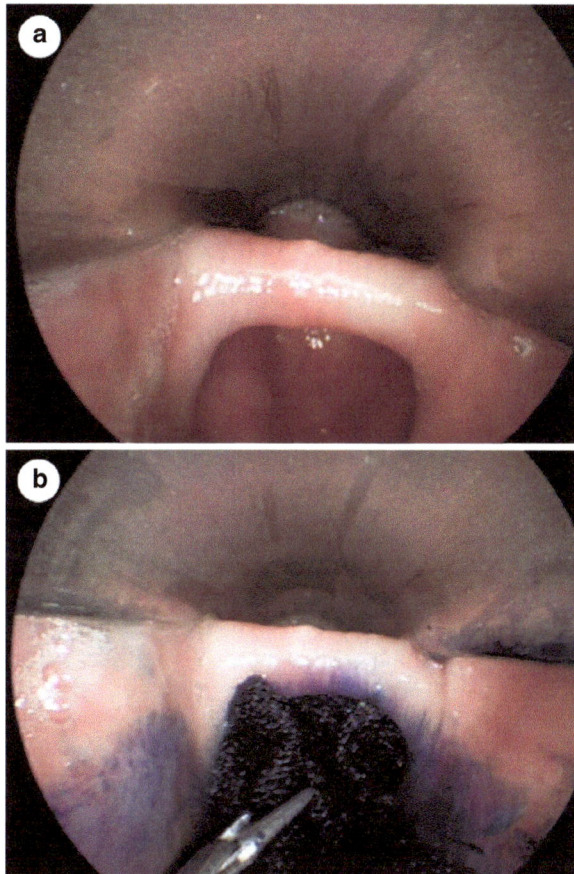

reached, the bougie should be easily palpable and often the sac itself due to the packing. Gentle staining from the methylene blue can be helpful to identify the sac. Using gentle finger dissection, it may be further delineated as it comes free from soft tissue attachments (Fig. 5.5). It may be necessary to retract the lateral aspect of the thyroid lobe medially in order to gain exposure.

Large diverticula may be paradoxically difficult to find. This is especially true in older male patients with low-lying larynges. The sac can settle into the upper mediastinum beyond the lordotic changes of the spine. Gentle manipulation of the laryngotracheal complex and bougie can "deliver" the sac into the operative field; again, care should be taken not to place traction on the RLN. The attachments between the sac and esophagus all the way up to the neck of the sac must be cleared. Often, this fascia over the expanding sac has become invested in the CP muscle itself. If not cleared up to the neck of the sac, this could lead to symptomatic failure.

Fig. 5.5 Intraoperative photo of a Zenker diverticulum (Z) protruding between the left inferior constrictor (IC) and cricopharyngeal muscle (CP). Note the Army Navy retractor on the left side of the image is behind the posterior thyroid ala, safely away from the cricothyroid joint and recurrent laryngeal nerve. Thyroid lobe (T)

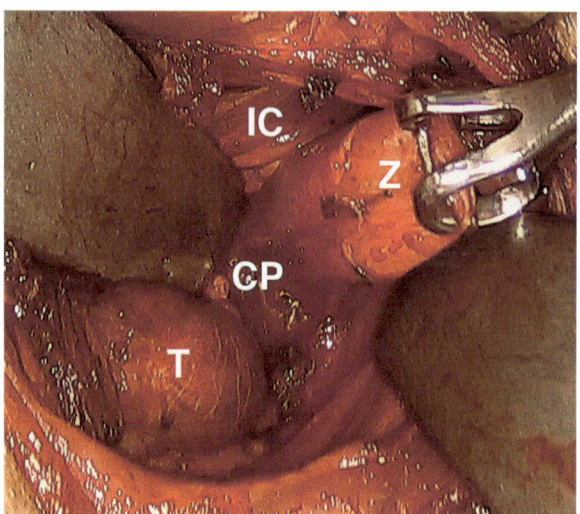

The methylene blue packing is removed by a non-scrubbed operating room staff member. It is imperative that the ETT must be kept in place as the packing is removed transorally. If accidental extubation occurs, it can be difficult to re-intubate an airway in which the pharynx has been colored with methylene blue and the larynx is often low-lying.

Now that the sac is fully exposed and the packing has been removed, the sac should be resected; this can be done using an enteral stapler or sharply with concomitant repair. The stapler resection can be easy and rapid, but the surgeon must be familiar with the various sizes of staplers in order to choose the appropriate one. The stapler automatically closes the hypopharyngeal defect (Fig. 5.6). The authors typically use a 45 mm blue load for an Ethicon ENDOPATH® ETS Articulating Linear Cutters (Ethicon, Cincinnati, OH). A single firing of the stapler is ideal. If multiple firings are required, careful note must be made to ensure staple lines overlap and there is no gap between staple lines. Alternatively, one may also resect the sac sharply over a clamp. The resulting hypopharyngeal defect is repaired using an imbricating suture with a 3-0 Vicryl on a small tapered (CV-23) needle.

Once the defect is repaired, a CP myotomy should be performed. A no. 15 blade can be used to feather through the muscle, or a sharp tenotomy scissors is used to dissect the plane between the muscle itself and the mucosa and allow for sharp transection of the muscle. This plane can be obscured in patients with previous dilation or other surgical procedures in the region such as anterior spine surgery, prior ZD repair, or carotid endarterectomy. The entirety of the CP muscle should be incised extending all the way from the proximal cervical esophagus to the neck of the sac. Care should be taken, however, not to extend

Fig. 5.6 Post-diverticulectomy and cricopharyngeal myotomy. The staple line is visible (Z), and only esophageal mucosa (E) remains post-myotomy.

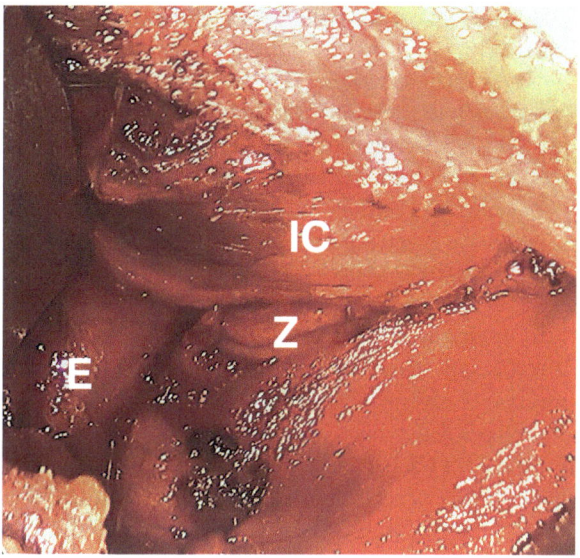

this too superiorly as the inferior constrictor is superior to the CP and plays a role in pharyngeal clearance.

Once the myotomy is completed, the bougie is removed. If one wishes to place a feeding tube, it should be placed carefully at this point. When passing the tube, ensure the diverticulectomy site is reinforced with digital pressure to prevent accidental perforation of the staple or suture line. Again, care should be taken not to dislodge the endotracheal tube. The surgical site is inspected for possible tears in the esophageal or hypopharyngeal mucosa. The surgical wound should then be copiously irrigated, and a dependent drain should be placed in the paraesophageal space. The omohyoid muscle should be reapproximated. A layered closure should be performed next with a 3-0 Vicryl for the platysmal/dermal layer and a 5-0 nylon for the skin. The drain is then secured with a stitch. Antibiotic ointment is applied. Next fluffs and a light elastic mesh dressing are placed.

The patient is then returned to the anesthesia team for emergence. It is important that positive pressure be avoided during wakeup. If positive pressure is needed (due to obstruction or neuromuscular weakness), it would be preferable for the patient to be re-intubated and then reevaluated for another extubation attempt.

Surgical Options

It should be noted that the preferred method of the authors is the diverticulectomy and myotomy (or myectomy) which happens to be the most common in practice [5], yet several other techniques for open procedures exist. Similar to endoscopic vs. open repair, solid evidence in favor of one approach over another is lacking.

Three main techniques are used—resection, inversion, and suspension. Resection (previously described) is the only technique which violates the mucosa. Inversion involves invagination of the mucosa into the esophageal lumen and oversewing of this inverted tissue. Diverticulopexy involves suturing the sac superiorly in a nondependent position, often to the prevertebral fascia or posterior pharyngeal wall.

Both the inversion and suspension techniques have a lower theoretical risk of leak because the mucosa is not entered. Mantsopoulos et al. [28] retrospectively compared outcomes of diverticulectomy with myotomy to the inversion technique. Fifty-four patients were included, only fourteen of whom (25.9%) underwent diverticulum inversion. Hospital times were significantly shorter for patients who underwent inversion, (8.9 days for inversion vs. 11 days for diverticulectomy). No significant differences were noted with respect to duration of operation, complication rates, or recurrence rates. From their own experience, the authors recommended the inversion procedure specifically for smaller diverticula. Others have also shown shorter time to oral intake as well as decreased complications for inversion rather than resection [29].

Diverticulopexy has been investigated as an alternative to resection as well. Greene et al. [30] retrospectively reviewed their series. Of open transcervical cases, 74% of these subjects (50 patients) underwent diverticulopexy, and 26% underwent diverticulectomy (18 patients). Complete resolution of symptoms occurred more often with diverticulopexy than diverticulectomy, but this was not found to be significant. Complication rates were not subdivided by the type of open technique. Simic et al. [31] compared resection with suspension (both with myotomy) in 50 patients. Eleven percent of suspension patients and 14% of diverticulectomy patients had recurrence of dysphagia; all patients were then symptom-free within 1 year of surgery. No pharyngocutaneous fistulas were observed.

Of note, when diverticulopexy or inversion is performed, the pouch itself is not removed, leaving behind poorly functional hypopharyngeal tissue. Secondly, there have been case reports of carcinoma arising in a long-standing pouch [32, 33], so one must take this into consideration when performing inversion and suspension which do not remove the pouch in its entirety.

Perioperative Care

Decisions about postoperative feeding are best made preoperatively based on the patient's swallowing status. Most patients fall somewhere between clearly needing a feeding tube preoperatively and clearly not needing one. Options for postoperative care include a G-tube, a nasogastric feeding tube, or a short period of nothing by mouth without a feeding tube. Some patient characteristics or comorbidities which may prompt enteral feeding include severe oropharyngeal dysphagia, extreme malnutrition, or extensive prior cervical surgery. If a feeding tube is to be placed after leaving the OR, interventional radiology placement is recommended, as blind

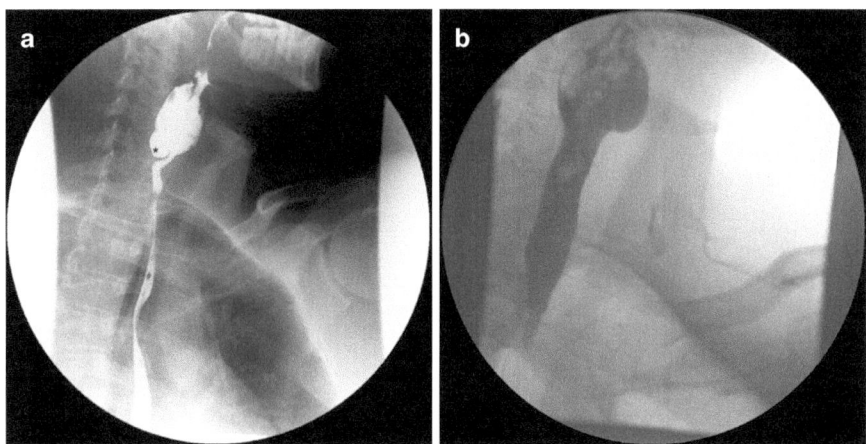

Fig. 5.7 (**a**) Preoperative barium swallow with small Zenker diverticulum seen posteriorly (asterisk). (**b**) Same patient, postoperatively, showing interval resolution of diverticulum on barium swallow

and even endoscopic placement of a feeding tube can be difficult in a patient with a recent open repair.

It is preferred, for patients with normal pharyngeal function, to avoid a feeding tube altogether. NPO status is kept for 1–2 days, while maintenance intravenous fluids are administered. A modified barium swallow or barium esophagram is performed on the first or second postoperative day. MBS is used for patients with significant preoperative dysfunction to insure there is no aspiration postoperatively as diet usually is heavily weighted toward liquids initially. If there is good outflow and no leak, the NG tube may be removed if present, and the patient can then be started on clear liquid diet (Fig. 5.7). For patients with a G-tube, there is less urgency to radiographically test the hypopharyngeal repair.

Diet is gradually advanced from clear to full liquids over the first week. Most patients are seen in the office roughly 1 week postoperatively. If they are doing well and progressing appropriately, diet is advanced to puree, soft, and then normal diet over the next couple of weeks. For patients with prolonged periods of NPO prior to surgery, speech pathology and nutritional consultation are utilized as needed.

Patients should all be given ample options for antiemetics, and any potential nausea should be acted on quickly; postoperative emesis should be avoided especially in open cases so as not to stress the newly repaired diverticulectomy site.

All patients are given antibiotics for the first week following surgery. Ampicillin/sulbactam is preferred, though a combination of cefazolin and metronidazole is also used. Clindamycin can be considered in the penicillin-allergic population.

The drain should be removed after oral intake has started and prior to discharge from the hospital. The drain is not there only to avoid hematoma, but rather to allow egress in order to reduce the risk of mediastinitis if there is a leak. Sutures should be removed at 1 week.

Fig. 5.8 Transcervical air seen on computed tomography on postoperative day 10 after starting CPAP on post-operative day 5 for central sleep apnea

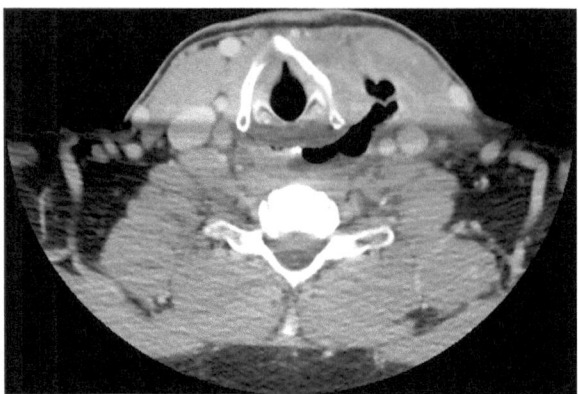

Once the patient leaves the hospital, many standard instructions apply. Effort should be made to avoid strenuous activity or heavy lifting for 14 days. Antiplatelet and anticoagulant therapy should be avoided for 1 week (as long as this is permissible with respect to other comorbidities). For patients with obstructive sleep apnea, it is important not to use any positive pressure device, such as continuous positive airway pressure (CPAP), to avoid air expression through the pharyngotomy closure which can create crepitus, destabilize the closure, and lead to infection (Fig. 5.8). For the same reason, positive pressure ventilation should be avoided upon emergence from anesthesia.

At the first postoperative visit, flexible fiber-optic laryngoscopy should be performed to assess for vocal fold motion, pharyngeal edema, hematoma, and residual pharyngeal pooling.

Complications

Open ZD surgery carries with it both short-term and long-term risks. Shortly after surgery, RLN injury, hematoma, perforation or pharyngocutaneous fistula, or mediastinitis may occur. In the long term, the major risk is persistent dysphagia or lack of symptomatic improvement.

Two of these complications are major distinguishing features between endoscopic and open surgery. RLN injury is reported to occur in 0–5% [4, 5, 8, 34] of open ZD cases. Because of this, vocal fold motion should be evaluated preoperatively; this is particularly pertinent if there is a preexisting immobility on the right (nonoperative side). Additionally, a unilateral RLN injury in and of itself reduces pulmonary protection and effective cough and would prove to be a significant concern in a fragile patient with an already dysfunctional swallow. Hematoma is another complication seen only with open repair which occurs roughly at 1–2.2% [4, 5]. As is always true in the head and neck, hematomas should be identified and treated early due to the potential for airway compromise.

Pharyngocutaneous fistula is a potential feared complication. Reported rates range from 0 to 8.3% [3–5, 31, 34]. If leaks occur early, they are typically recognized by change in drain output or with postsurgical swallow imaging. Small leaks should heal quickly if flow through the esophagus is not obstructed; patients should be treated with enteral feeding and packing to the fistula site until output ceases.

Leaks can occur in a delayed fashion as well. These arguably are of more concern because drains typically have been removed and oral intake has been initiated. While all patients with leaks are at risk for mediastinitis, this population is more concerning because of possible delay in identification which can allow maturation of an infection.

Mediastinitis is a potentially fatal complication caused by bacteria in saliva or food leaking through the esophageal or hypopharyngeal perforation and infecting the surrounding soft tissues. As the fascial planes of the neck are connected to the mediastinum, this can cause infection of the chest which can quickly become fatal. These planes are disturbed during the dissection of the pouch. This is generally not experienced during endoscopic procedures which may explain, in part, why mediastinitis is a rare complication of ESD. Physicians should be alert for any of the classic symptoms of this infection, namely, fever, tachycardia, and chest or upper back pain. If present, one should obtain a white blood cell count to assess for potential infection (though notably in the postoperative period an elevated white blood cell count can be normal, a severe leukocytosis is indicative of something more nefarious). If the clinical picture is concerning for hypopharyngeal leak or mediastinitis, all feeds (oral or otherwise) must be stopped, and antibiotics should be continued and likely broadened.

If mediastinitis is suspected in the immediate post-op period, typically the quality of the drain output changes. If drainage worsens, returning to the operating room for wound washout and re-draining is prudent. If it is beyond the first couple of days postoperatively and the drain has been removed already, CT imaging with contrast is helpful in identifying the presence and extent of the process. Typically, mediastinitis can be managed via transcervical drainage; however, thoracic surgery consultation is advised in the event that infection advances.

Mediastinitis and hypopharyngeal fistulas typically improve with drainage and time. Reduction of salivary flow with use of scopolamine can help slow output. If the hypopharyngeal defect is small, patience and wound care often result in resolution. If more substantial, transcervical exploration with primary closure and reinforcement with a local or regional rotational flap is recommended. Once drainage ceases from the neck, esophageal imaging is repeated, and, if negative, oral intake is initiated.

Conclusions

Open Zenker diverticulum surgery is the most definitive treatment available for ZD. Though operating times tend to be longer, lengths of stay are longer, and complications are of a different ilk than those encountered with endoscopic procedures, overall the procedure is safe and effective. Open surgery, however, is not the appropriate choice for repair in every patient. Given this, surgeons should be competent in both open and endoscopic treatments.

Acknowledgments   The authors have no relevant disclosures or declarations.

References

1. Hillel AT, Flint PW. Evolution of endoscopic surgical therapy for Zenker's diverticulum. Laryngoscope. 2009;119:39–44.
2. Collard JM, Otte JB, Kestens PJ. Endoscopic stapling technique of esophagodiverticulostomy for Zenker's diverticulum. Ann Thorac Surg. 1993;56:573–6.
3. Wirth D, Kern B, Guenin MO, Montali I, Peterli R, Ackermann C, von Flue M. Outcome and quality of life after open surgery versus endoscopic stapler-assisted esophagodiverticulostomy for Zenker's diverticulum. Dis Esophagus. 2006;19:294–8.
4. Verdonck J, Morton RP. Systematic review on treatment of Zenker's diverticulum. Eur Arch Otorhinolaryngol. 2015;272:3095–107.
5. Yuan Y, Zhao YF, Hu Y, Chen LQ. Surgical treatment of Zenker's diverticulum. Dig Surg. 2013;30:207–18.
6. Albers DV, Kondo A, Bernardo WM, Sakai P, Moura RN, Silva GL, Ide E, Tomishige T, de Moura EG. Endoscopic versus surgical approach in the treatment of Zenker's diverticulum: systematic review and meta-analysis. Endosc Int Open. 2016;4:E678–86.
7. Chang CW, Burkey BB, Netterville JL, Courey MS, Garrett CG, Bayles SW. Carbon dioxide laser endoscopic diverticulotomy versus open diverticulectomy for Zenker's diverticulum. Laryngoscope. 2004;114:519–27.
8. Chang CY, Payyapilli RJ, Scher RL. Endoscopic staple diverticulostomy for Zenker's diverticulum: review of literature and experience in 159 consecutive cases. Laryngoscope. 2003;113:957–65.
9. Counter PR, Hilton ML, Baldwin DL. Long-term follow-up of endoscopic stapled diverticulotomy. Ann R Coll Surg Engl. 2002;84:89–92.
10. Raut VV, Primrose WJ. Long-term results of endoscopic stapling diverticulotomy for pharyngeal pouches. Otolaryngol Head Neck Surg. 2002;127:225–9.
11. Seth R, Rajasekaran K, Lee WT, et al. Patient reported outcomes in endoscopic and open transcervical treatment for Zenker's diverticulum. Laryngoscope. 2014;124:119–25.
12. Schoeff S, Freeman M, Daniero J. Voice outcomes in surgical repair of Zenker's diverticulum. Dysphagia. 2017;32:678–82.
13. Leung JM, Dzankic S. Relative importance of preoperative health status versus intraoperative factors in predicting postoperative adverse outcomes in geriatric surgical patients. J Am Geriatr Soc. 2001;49:1080–5.
14. Turrentine FE, Wang H, Simpson VB, Jones RS. Surgical risk factors, morbidity, and mortality in elderly patients. J Am Coll Surg. 2006;203:865–77.
15. Bloom JD, Bleier BS, Mirza N, Chalian AA, Thaler ER. Factors predicting endoscopic exposure of Zenker's diverticulum. Ann Otol Rhinol Laryngol. 2010;119:736–41.
16. Koch M, Mantsopoulos K, Velegrakis S, Iro H, Zenk J. Endoscopic laser-assisted diverticulotomy versus open surgical approach in the treatment of Zenker's diverticulum. Laryngoscope. 2011;121:2090–4.
17. Rizzetto C, Zaninotto G, Costantini M, Bottin R, Finotti E, Zanatta L, Guirroli E, Ceolin M, Nicoletti L, Ruol A, Ancona E. Zenker's diverticula: feasibility of a tailored approach based on diverticulum size. J Gastrointest Surg. 2008;12:2057–64.
18. Cook RD, Huang PC, Richstmeier WJ, Scher RL. Endoscopic staple-assisted esophagodiverticulostomy: an excellent treatment of choice for Zenker's diverticulum. Laryngoscope. 2000;110:2020–5.
19. Casso C, Lalam M, Ghosh S, Timms M. Endoscopic stapling diverticulotomy: an audit of difficulties, outcome, and patient satisfaction. Otolaryngol Head Neck Surg. 2006;134:288–93.
20. Van Abel KM, Tombers NM, Krein KA, Moore EJ, Price DL, Kasperbauer JL, Hinni ML, Lott DG, Ekbom DC. Short-term quality-of-life outcomes following transoral diverticulotomy for Zenker's Diverticulum: a prospective single-group study. Otolaryngol Head Neck Surg 2016; 154:322-327.

21. van Overbeek JJ. Meditation on the pathogenesis of hypopharyngeal (Zenker's) diverticulum and a report of endoscopic treatment in 545 patients. Ann Otol Rhinol Laryngol. 1994;103:178–85.
22. Rubesin SE, Levine MS. Killian-Jamieson diverticula: radiographic findings in 16 patients. AJR Am J Roentgenol. 2001;177:85–9.
23. Kim DC, Hwang JJ, Lee WS, Lee SA, Kim YH, Chee HK. Surgical treatment of Killian-Jamieson diverticulum. Korean J Thorac Cardiovasc Surg. 2012;45:272–4.
24. Pinto JA, Marquis VB, de Godoy LB, Magri EN, Brunoro MV. Bilateral hypopharyngeal diverticulum. Otolaryngol Head Neck Surg. 2009;141:144–5.
25. Clay B. Congenital lateral pharyngeal diverticulum. Br J Radiol. 1972;45:863–5.
26. Naunheim M, Langerman A. Pharyngoceles: a photo-anatomic study and novel management. Laryngoscope. 2013;123:1632–8.
27. Weisberg NK, Spengler DM, Netterville JL. Stretch-induced nerve injury as a cause of paralysis secondary to the anterior cervical approach. Otolaryngol Head Neck Surg. 1997;116:317–26.
28. Mantsopoulos K, Psychogios G, Kunzel J, Zenk J, Iro H, Koch M. Evaluation of the different transcervical approaches for Zenker diverticulum. Otolaryngol Head Neck Surg. 2012;146:725–9.
29. Morton RP, Bartley JR. Inversion of Zenker's diverticulum: the preferred option. Head Neck. 1993;15:253–6.
30. Greene CL, McFadden PM, Oh DS, Chang EJ, Hagen JA. Long-term outcome of the treatment of Zenker's diverticulum. Ann Thorac Surg. 2015;100:975–8.
31. Simic A, Radovanovic N, Stojakov D, Bjelović M, Kotarac M, Sabljak P, Skrobić O, Pesko P. Surgical experience of the national institution in the treatment of Zenker's diverticula. Acta Chir Iugosl. 2009;56:25–33.
32. Bowdler DA, Stell PM. Carcinoma arising in posterior pharyngeal pulsion diverticulum (Zenker's diverticulum). Br J Surg. 1987;74:561–3.
33. Nanson EM. Carcinoma in a long-standing pharyngeal diverticulum. Br J Surg. 1976;63:417–9.
34. Feeley MA, Righi PD, Weisberger EC, Hamaker RC, Spahn TJ, Radpour S, Wynne MK. Zenker's diverticulum: analysis of surgical complications from diverticulectomy and cricopharyngeal myotomy. Laryngoscope. 1999;109:858–61.

Endoscopic Staple Diverticulostomy for Zenker Diverticulum

William J. Richtsmeier and Richard L. Scher

Introduction

To grasp the impact that the introduction of endoscopic staple diverticulostomy (ESD) had for the treatment of Zenker diverticulum (ZD), one needs to understand the historical reputation of endoscopic surgery for ZD. It was only with technical advancements reported in the 1980s that the clinical acceptance of endoscopic treatment began to spread globally.

The fear of and hesitancy to utilize endoscopic surgery for ZD started as soon as endoscopic surgery was first reported by Mosher in 1917 [1], with early recognition that endoscopic approaches had unreasonably high risks for significant morbidity and death. This view was placated to some extent by Dohlman and Mattsson's report "The Endoscopic Operation for Hypopharyngeal Diverticula," [2] but endoscopic approaches still never became popular in the United States due to concerns for unacceptably high rates of mediastinitis that resulted from the "sutureless" approach to dividing the common wall between the diverticulum and esophagus. This fear was partly true because the primary population of patients with ZD, the elderly, often had multiple comorbidities and poor performance status placing them in higher-risk categories for surgery. Together with the fact that perioperative supportive care was inconsistent and lacking today's expertise and medical advances, many surgeons considered endoscopic treatment of ZD too risky for widespread clinical adoption.

W. J. Richtsmeier (✉)
Division of Otolaryngology, Bassett Medical Center, Cooperstown, NY, USA
e-mail: william.richtsmeier@bassett.org

R. L. Scher
ENT Procedure Innovation and Development, Olympus Corporation, Tokyo, Japan

Division of Head and Neck Surgery and Communication Sciences, Department of Surgery, Duke University, Durham, NC, USA
e-mail: richard.scher@olympus.com

Similarly, because of the perceived risks of all surgical approaches, many internists would not refer patients for surgery out of genuine concern for their overall survival, as well as poor patient acceptance of the procedures. Surgery was often considered only when serious sequelae related to the ZD occurred, such as recurrent aspiration pneumonia, or significant weight loss with malnutrition. Referred patients were often weak, poorly nourished, depressed, and quite elderly, with little reserve with which to deal with surgical stress and potential complications. Open surgical approaches with diverticulectomy, diverticulopexy, or cricopharyngeal myotomy were perceived as quite invasive, with a neck incision and several days with uncomfortable NG tube feeding and hospitalization.

Following Dohlman and Mattsson's report of endoscopic treatment using diathermy to divide the common wall between the diverticulum and esophagus, further technological refinements were made that reduced the risk of surgical morbidity and led to greater adoption and use of endoscopic treatment for ZD. In 1984, van Overbeek and colleagues introduced the use of the operating microscope and carbon dioxide (CO_2) laser to endoscopic treatment of ZD [3]. Complication rates and symptom resolution were demonstrated to be equal to or improved over historical outcomes for open treatment approaches. Subsequent independent reports by Martin-Hirsch and Newbegin [4] in England and Collard and associates [5] in Belgium in 1993 introduced an endoscopic stapling technique for performing an esophagodiverticulostomy for ZD. The technique was refined and introduced in the United States by Scher and Richtsmeier [6]. This approach created a "sutured" closure of the mucosal edges, with the endoscopic staples sealing the mucosal and muscular cut created during the division of the common wall. The reported outcomes for this endoscopic staple esophagodiverticulostomy (ESD) demonstrated improved morbidity and mortality compared to other endoscopic and open approaches, as well as rapid convalescence, reduced operative time, and shortened hospital stay [7, 8]. These reports of the application of surgical endoscopic staplers for endoscopic treatment of ZD prompted a quick acceptance of the safety and efficacy by the endoscopic approach and led to widespread adoption of this method as a primary treatment for patients with ZD.

Diagnosis and Patient Selection

Patient history alone may raise suspicion for ZD. The predominant symptom is progressive dysphagia, often with regurgitation of food even hours after a meal. Other symptoms include frequent belching, hypopharyngeal mucus collection, halitosis, choking, coughing, hoarseness, globus pharyngeus, weight loss, and recurrent respiratory infections. Patients may experience symptoms for weeks to many years before diagnosis, with little correlation between severity of symptoms and ZD size. Physical findings may include mucus pooling in the hypopharynx that initially clears with swallowing and then recurs and in some cases emaciation or dehydration as sequelae of the ZD. However, it is more often the case that patients are without any specific findings on physical examination.

Diagnosis is confirmed by contrast barium radiography, which can also define the size and position of the ZD. It is important to review the study looking for several important features. The radiologic study needs to have a good lateral view to determine the presence of a pouch, its anatomic orientation with the larynx, and its delayed or lack of emptying of contrast material with repeated swallow attempts. A modified barium swallow using contrast materials of varying consistency with cineradiographic review typically gives a better estimation of the degree of severity of the dysphagia. Unfortunately, in some communities the lower esophagus is not critically examined with a modified barium swallow study. A second contrast study may be required to complete the evaluation. Anterior-posterior views are also necessary to determine laterality of the ZD. The depth of the pouch usually can be estimated by comparing it to the size of the patient's vertebral bodies. If the depth of the pouch in the unexpanded state, that is, the relaxed portion of the swallow, is the length of a vertebral body, then there is usually enough depth to perform an adequate cricopharyngeal myotomy by ESD. It is also important to make sure that there is no distal esophageal obstruction seen in the study and to assess for other functional and anatomic abnormalities that can affect swallow function, such as esophageal reflux, hiatal hernia, or esophageal dysmotility. Such factors may continue to adversely affect swallowing function after successful ESD, and patients should be counseled about this possibility preoperatively and steps made to address other pathologies.

In addition, the cervical spine can usually be assessed with the lateral radiographic view to assess for any appearance of degenerative findings suggestive of arthritis. Osteophytes present on the anterior vertebral bodies are of particular concern as they may contribute to the dysphagia and present an additional difficulty in placing the laryngoscope during endoscopic exposure of the ZD. Inability to satisfactorily visualize the post-cricoid space during rigid endoscopy has been reported to be as high as 30% [9] but as low as 4% in large series [8]. It is worth having a conversation with the patient as to whether they want a transcervical myotomy and possible diverticulectomy performed if endoscopic visualization of the ZD and esophagus can't be adequately accomplished to allow ESD.

While ESD does not require antibiotics, it is worth considering if you would want antibiotics given preoperatively should there be a complication such as a pharyngeal laceration. Many surgeons will give a preoperative dose of IV steroids to minimize laryngeal edema from endoscope pressure and local periesophageal swelling which may interfere with immediate postoperative swallowing resulting in a delay in discharge.

Endoscopic Staple Diverticulostomy Technique

Endoscopic Staplers

Use of the ESD approach to treatment requires an understanding of the Endo GIA 30 stapler design, function, and limitations (Medtronic Minneapolis MN). The concept of using the staplers designed for laparoscopic surgery for treating ZD endoscopically involved the realization that they were well suited for this use. They have a mechanism that simultaneously performs both the myotomy and securing of the mucosa of the esophageal and diverticular common wall division. This feature significantly, if not almost completely, negates the potential for salivary leakage and the associated fear of postoperative mediastinitis. The stapler creates a conduit from the pouch into the superior esophagus, an esophagodiverticulostomy. Additionally, the stapler shaft design and length allow instrumentation through the Weerda laryngoscope, along with telescopic visualization (discussed below) while having appropriate dimensions of the staple cartridge and anvil to engage the common wall for treatment.

Knowing how the staplers work and their limitations is critical to a good outcome [10] and is illustrated in Fig. 6.1. The cartridge holds staples of varying length whose choice depends on the tissue being treated. We have used the thin-vascular load that comes with the Endo GIA 30 stapler. With activation of the stapler, the incorporated knife is pushed forward cutting the tissue enclosed between the blades of the stapler and anvil. Simultaneously, the staples are advanced into the tissue on each side of the cut, with compression of the staples sealing each side of the mucosal and muscular division [11]. Complications such as leaks from the staple line can occur from incorrect staple length choice [12], poor staple conformation, or stapler malfunction, all of which are uncommon. It can be seen in Fig. 6.1 that the staples extend further than the myotomy created by the knife blade by two staples. This

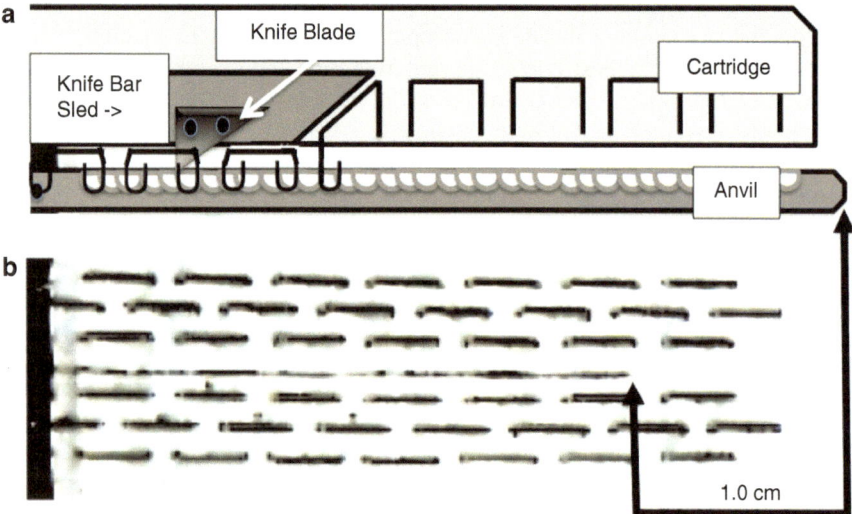

Fig. 6.1 Diagram of the mechanism of an endoscopic surgical stapler part way through being "fired" (**a**) (above) and a photo (**b**) (below) of the result of firing a GIA 30 stapler into a paper towel in the same orientation of the stapler entering from left to right (Bottom right arrows indicate the obligate residual pouch due to stapler configuration)

provides security in wound closure. This safety feature also limits the length of the myotomy that can be achieved, but without significance for clinical outcome of symptom relief in the majority of cases.

Other limitations of the staplers for treatment of ZD include the lack of maneuverability of the device in the sagittal plane (some move in the coronal plane), the extension of the anvil beyond the staple placement in tissue, and the size limitations of the instrument shaft. None of these represent a significant impediment to successful use, but it is important to be aware of them. The staplers available for endoscopic use always leave, at least, a 1.0 cm inferior common wall after stapler activation. In the postoperative patient, this can be mistaken for a residual or recurrent diverticulum despite an adequate myotomy [10]. This will be discussed further in the technique section.

Endoscopic Visualization

A second important innovation and technical feature of ESD is the addition of telescopic inspection during all parts of the procedure. This aspect is important for assessment of the pouch for cleaning and measurement of depth, control of proper placement of the stapler, assessment of adequate myotomy, and inspection for possible pharyngeal laceration or other problems at completion of the ESD. Coupling of the telescope to camera and monitoring systems allows intraoperative visualization for the surgeon and operating room staff while providing image capture and recording capability of the surgeon's activity for teaching and assessment.

Laryngoscopes for ESD

The choice of laryngoscope is important for proper exposure of the ZD and esophagus during ESD. The standard endoscope commonly used for this is the Weerda large laryngoscope (Karl Storz, Culver City, CA) (Fig. 6.2). This laryngoscope is a bivalve scope that allows adjustment of the proximal and distal apertures and is long enough to allow passage beyond the post-cricoid hypopharynx in most patients. The open bivalve design also allows space laterally for instruments to be used side by side. This is important during ESD when a telescope is placed alongside the stapler to ensure that the stapler is positioned and deployed accurately and safely. In some patients, the Weerda large laryngoscope is not long enough to provide exposure. In this situation, the Weerda diverticuloscope can be used. This scope is designed similar to the laryngoscope, but with an additional 6 cm of length to the blades. The disadvantage of this scope is that the longer blades can be torqued by arthritic changes in the cervical spine, or the larynx, making exposure difficult. For the majority of patients, the Weerda laryngoscope provides adequate exposure of the ZD and room for instrument manipulation. The authors have also occasionally

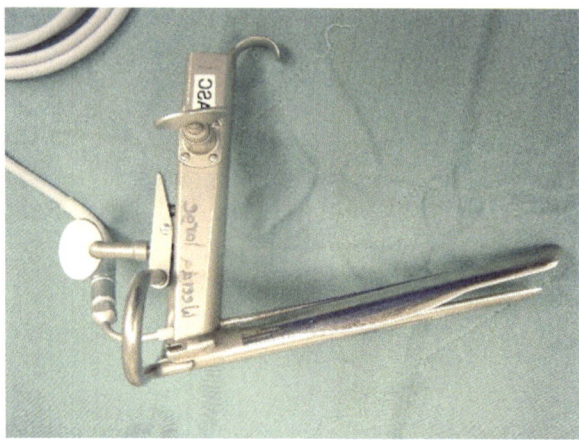

Fig. 6.2 The Weerda laryngoscope, with ability to adjust the distal and proximal apertures

performed this procedure using a Jako laryngoscope which also gives good elevation of the posterior aspect of the larynx and just enough room to perform the procedure.

The authors have found it is sometimes useful to pass the short Jesberg esophagoscope to view the esophagus and pouch prior to employing the laryngoscope. The Jesberg esophagoscope easily slides through the lingual sulcus rather than directly over the teeth the way a laryngoscope or diverticuloscope is usually positioned. Visualization of the unoperated esophagus provides an opportunity for endoscopic placement of a nasogastric (NG) tube in those cases where conversion to an open procedure is felt necessary due to inadequate endoscopic exposure. In routine ESD, a NG tube is not utilized. If there are concerns that it may be too difficult to visualize the common wall with the laryngoscope or diverticuloscope, an open myotomy may be necessary.

Operative Technique

The patient is administered a general anesthetic with a medium-sized endotracheal tube. Generally, it is useful to have the tube secured to the skin overlying the mandible or left cheek. The patient should have complete muscle relaxation provided by the anesthesiologist, with the understanding that there will be a very short period of time between the end of dividing and stapling the common wall segment and completion of the procedure. This helps to ensure that emergence from anesthesia is not excessively long.

The patient should have dentures removed if present and a maxillary tooth guard placed for patients with teeth. The head is positioned in the "sniffing" position with slight neck extension and head elevation, as is a routine for transoral rigid endoscopic procedures [13]. Having the patient on an operating table with a side rail that will support a device such as the Karl Storz, Lubeck chest support (part # 8585S), allows for over-the-chest support for the laryngoscope suspension system. A Mayo stand can be substituted but is less secure and does not move with the patient should table height or angulation change after the scope is in position.

The scope is introduced in the usual way for laryngoscopy and directed into the hypopharynx and post-cricoid region. The scope is maneuvered behind the larynx and elevated to visualize the esophageal introitus and the diverticulum. The pouch is usually easily seen as in Fig. 6.3. At this point the scope is secured with the suspension system. The Weerda laryngoscope is then appropriately opened proximally and distally to give enough space within the laryngoscope lumen to allow the stapler and the telescope to be placed simultaneously while adequately exposing the surgical area.

The Weerda laryngoscope or diverticuloscope should be placed with the blades just proximal to the esophageal and diverticular openings. Placement of the blades inside the esophageal lumen and into the pouch is not required to provide good surgical exposure and risks injury to the mucosa when the blades are distended to allow adequate exposure.

The pouch is examined to remove any food debris and to assess for adequate depth and size for ESD (Fig. 6.3). Debris often consists of undigested food, pills, and occasionally substances such as barium from previous contrast studies. If a laceration of the pharynx should occur during the procedure, one would not want the contents of the pouch to contaminate the neck.

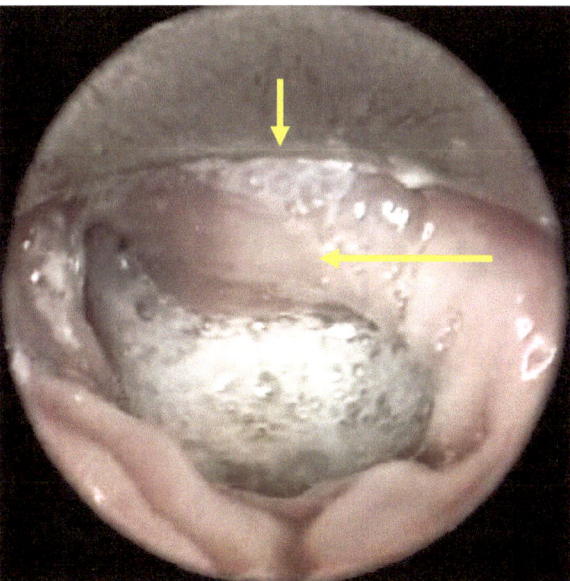

Fig. 6.3 Endoscopic view of ZD. Mucus bubbles are seen in the ZD posterior to the cricopharyngeal wall (long arrow). Esophageal opening is just posterior to the flange of the Weerda laryngoscope (short arrow)

The pouch should be thoroughly examined to ensure that it is indeed intact and does not contain a neoplasm [14, 15]. The pouch depth should be estimated to ensure a 2.0–2.5 cm depth which would allow for an adequate myotomy using the standard Endo GIA 30 stapler.

If the pouch or, more likely, the esophagus is difficult to visualize, it can be identified by carefully palpating the folds of mucosa with a spatula (Figs. 6.4 and 6.5). One has to be careful not to press too firmly when palpating and cause a laceration. Usually the mucosa of the pouch can be seen to "tent" in with slight pressure. Next the esophagus is explored with the same instrument where it should freely pass into the upper esophagus with no tenting of the tissue or resistance indicating lumenal patency. This confirms proper positioning of the scope and the target for the stapling procedure.

Placement of Traction Sutures

The authors have routinely placed a traction suture in the lateral aspect of the common wall mucosa over the cricopharyngeus muscle as a means of helping to provide countertraction on the common wall during placement of the stapler. This is useful for smaller pouches, as additional tissue can be gently pulled into the stapler blades, and for larger pouches when more than one staple cartridge is going to be placed (Fig. 6.6). Given excellent exposure, two traction sutures, one on each side of the common wall, can be placed; however, one is often sufficient. The suture can be placed with the Endo Stitch Autosuture device (Medtronic). Becoming familiar with the Endo Stitch prior to the procedure is helpful so that the surgeon knows where the needle is at any given time and how it can be released. The stitch is placed by placing the jaw of the device containing the needle in the pouch and passing it

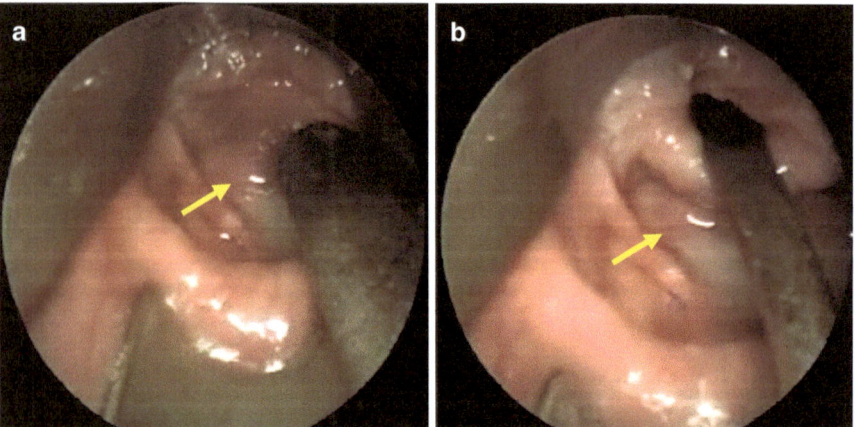

Fig. 6.4 The esophagus initially may be difficult to see (**a**) but can be identified with a spatula (**b**) using gentle probing. The spatula depresses the cricopharyngeal wall and exposes the esophageal lumen. Arrow, Zenker diverticulum

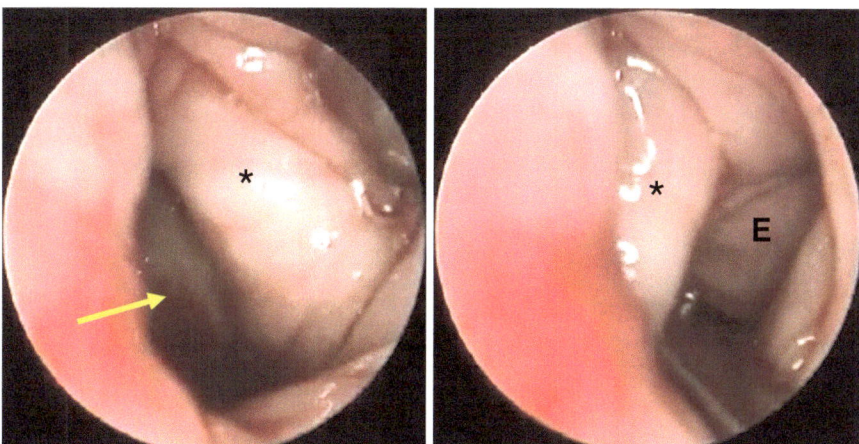

Fig. 6.5 Difficult to find esophagus in elderly patient with ZD. Diverticuloscope is pushed to one side by vertebral osteophyte. A large ZD (arrow) is seen on left; spatula is in upper right corner of image. Common wall between ZD and esophagus (asterisk). Esophagus (E) exposed by gentle pressure with the spatula in image on the right. When the esophageal lumen is pushed open, the ZD is no longer clearly visualized

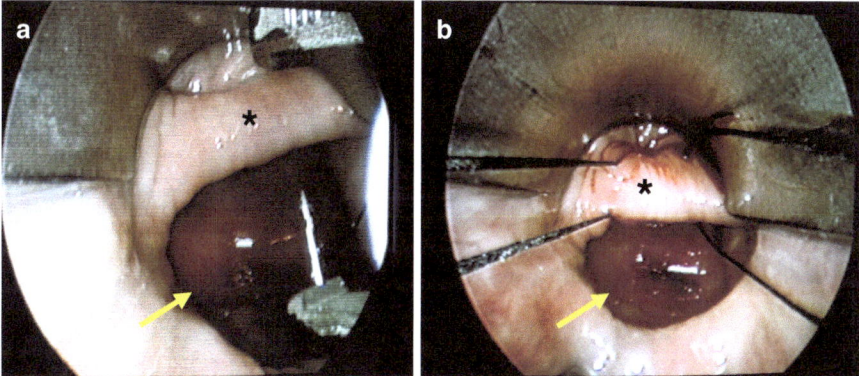

Fig. 6.6 Autosuture device used to place retraction sutures in common wall (asterisk) between esophagus and ZD (arrow). (**a**) The blade containing the needle is placed into the ZD, and then with device activation, the needle is passed to the opposite blade in the esophagus and withdrawn. (**b**) Bilateral retraction sutures have been placed. The sutures are placed as far lateral in the common wall as possible in order to allow room for placement of the Endo GIA stapler

into the esophagus. Retrieving a free needle can be more difficult than expected, and the Endo Stich resolves this issue by never completely letting go of it.

Passing from the pouch to the esophagus allows placement without risk of inadvertent injury to the esophageal mucosa. Traction sutures will eventually be removed, so whether they are absorbable or not is unimportant. If nonabsorbable suture is used, care should be taken to ensure all suture material is removed at the completion of the procedure in order to prevent inadvertent scar formation across the esophagodiverticulostomy. Suture can occasionally become caught in the staple line, but gentle traction is usually sufficient for removal. A "tag" such as a straight clamp is attached to both ends of the traction suture so that there is slight gravitational pull.

Employment of the Stapler

The stapler is then inspected to ensure that it is loaded with the proper cartridge. The thin-vascular load is recommended for the Endo GIA 30 stapler [16]. The cartridge-anvil complex of the GIA 30 rotates allowing it to be held in a position where either is positioned anteriorly to the diverticulum. In examining the stapler, it is easy to identify that the cartridge containing the staples protrudes slightly further than the anvil. As the length of the incision is limited by the depth that the stapler can enter the pouch, it is generally preferable to place the staple cartridge in the esophagus and the anvil in the pouch to maximize this relationship (Fig. 6.7). Occasionally, the opening to the esophagus is difficult to visualize or appears more anterior making it difficult to enter with the cartridge which is in a straight line with the shaft of the stapler. In such a case, an initial stapling can be carried out with the anvil in the esophagus, expecting less than maximum depth of penetration. This will be followed with a second stapling reversing the anvil/cartridge relationship [17]. The same care

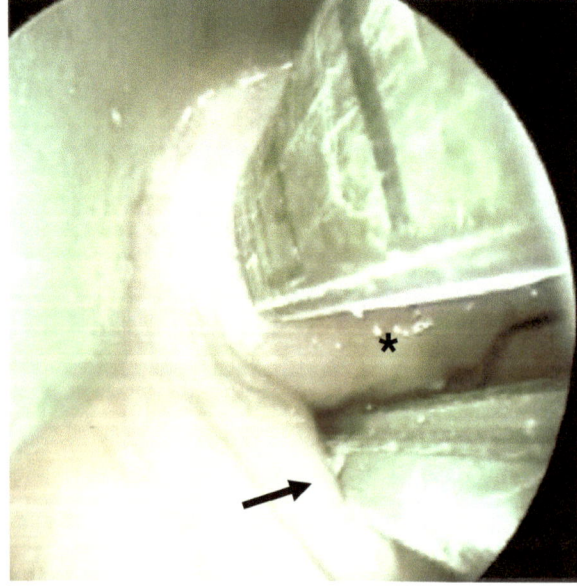

Fig. 6.7 The GIA 30 stapler has engaged the CP segment (asterisk). The traction suture can be seen at far right between the stapler jaws. Note the anvil is in the ZD pouch (arrow) and the cartridge is in the esophagus expecting a second stapling to maximize the depth of myotomy

must be used with placing the stapler during the second application as it can also produce a laceration at the apex of the pouch. The engagement of the stapler with the common wall is continuously visualized with the use of a telescope attached to a video monitoring system.

In engaging the stapler with the common wall, it is useful to place the partially opened stapler in such a manner that the opening is at the level of the muscle at rest and pull the traction suture lightly to help engage the common wall into the mouth of the stapler as much as possible. A series of short, light taps with the traction suture seems to work better than a steady pull. Care must be taken not to pull so hard that the anvil perforates the mucosa of the pouch. The pouch is usually much broader than the esophagus, and some tenting of the apex can occur which allows a few more millimeters of engagement. Once the stapler has satisfactorily engaged the common wall, the jaws are closed, and the stapler is activated which pushes the sled inside the cartridge that extrudes the staples and pushes the blade forward, cutting the mucosa. The stapler is opened, and the esophageal and diverticular mucosal closure that is stapled to the underlying muscle retracts away from the midline leaving a "V"-shaped incision (Fig. 6.8).

Even if the stapler engages the common wall to its full 30 mm depth, one can gain additional myotomy length with a second stapler placement through the apex of the V assuming there is additional pouch depth with which to work. In this case, bilateral retraction sutures are very helpful in allowing additional pouch to be

Fig. 6.8 Completed esophagodiverticulostomy. The Endo GIA 30 stapler has been "fired" and removed, revealing the "V"-shaped incision (arrows) and the staple secured mucosal margin. The traction suture is still present on the right. Pouch remnant (asterisk) visible below incision, and the additional depth of pouch is visible to accept a second stapling. Esophageal lumen (E)

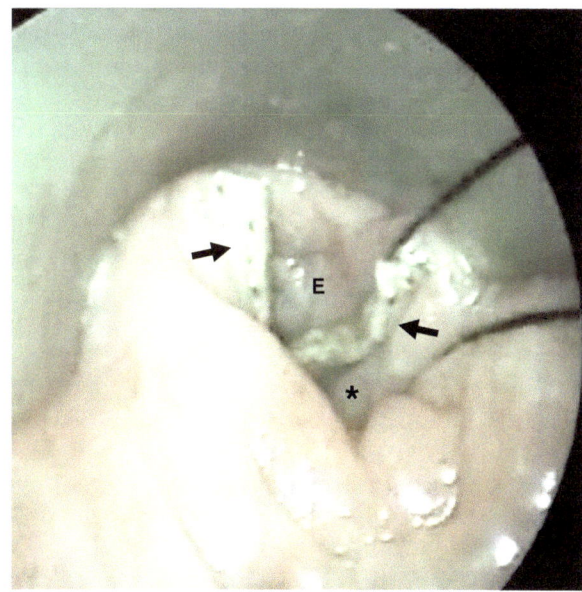

"pulled" into the jaws of the second stapler. Overlapping staples do not provide any postoperative complications. Some surgeons regularly extend the incision beyond that performed by the stapler using a scissor or laser. It should be remembered that the major goal is safety and the distal staples are there for that purpose. Extending the incision beyond the staple line increases the possibility of salivary leakage from the esophagodiverticulostomy.

At the completion of the common wall division, it is important to examine the pouch with the telescope and ensure that there is no laceration. Management of a laceration will be discussed under complications. Once an adequate esophagodiverticulostomy is created, the retraction sutures are removed. The laryngoscope is then withdrawn, and the patient awakened from anesthesia. A nasogastric tube is not placed unless a complication has occurred that will necessitate making the patient *nil per os* beyond 24 hours.

Postoperative Care

The patient is discharged home on the day of surgery after 3–4 hours of observation to assess for signs of complications. These include fever, chest or back pain, subcutaneous emphysema, hemoptysis, tachycardia, tachypnea, or respiratory distress. If any of these are present, immediate appropriate evaluation is initiated as described below. The patient is instructed to have only a clear liquid diet the night of surgery and advance as tolerated to a regular diet beginning the next day. The use of antibiotics on a routine basis before, during, or after surgery has been found to be unnecessary. During the postoperative period, no role for barium esophagography has been found except when evaluation of possible recurrence is necessary [18–20]. When performed in the asymptomatic patient, such radiographic studies usually reveal a residual diverticulum that does not retain barium and so has no clinical bearing on, or correlation with, outcome [19–22]. The procedure itself takes about 30 minutes to perform [7]. Compared with external approaches, ESD results in shorter hospital stay; shorter anesthesia times, which is important in the elderly or the medically infirm; and more rapid convalescence [8].

Outcomes

Endoscopic staple-assisted diverticulotomy has been shown to have consistent safety and efficacy. Outcomes of this technique have been studied since its inception in the early 1990s. In Collard's study from 1993, six patients were treated with this technique [5]. All patients had improvement or resolution in their complaints of dysphagia, although a small diverticular remnant was seen on follow-up MBSS. No patients had postoperative fevers or developed major complications. A larger study by Scher et al. evaluated 36 consecutive patients undergoing stapler-assisted Zenker diverticulotomy [22]. In this group, 72% of patients had complete improvement,

17% had some improvement, and 6% had no change in their symptoms, requiring revision surgery. The average hospital stay in this group was 1.3 days (range 1–4 days). Another study by Peracchia et al. reported on 105 patients undergoing this procedure in 1998, with a complete resolution of symptoms in 95% without significant morbidity or mortality [23]. A large study from Chang et al. evaluating 159 cases showed complete resolution of symptoms in 63%, partial improvement in 25%, and no change in 11% [7]. In this group, average hospital stay was 0.76 days, and average time to diet initiation (clear liquids) was 0.25 days. In the Barton et al. study evaluating 106 patients, 20 patients underwent a stapler-assisted diverticulotomy and experienced a significant average improvement in their Eating Assessment Tool-10 (EAT-10) score of 8 points [24]. A more recent larger study of over 300 patients further supports these results [8].

Complications

The common complications of the ESD approach are listed in Table 6.1. Major complications have been reported to occur in 5.6% of cases and minor complications as often as 9.3% [8]. Review of these potential complications is an important part of informed consent. Successful management of them requires appropriate recognition. In the previously mentioned study by Scher et al. evaluating 36 patients undergoing endoscopic stapler-assisted diverticulotomy, a 14% overall complication rate was reported: 6% dental injury, 3% postoperative fever, 3% transient vocal fold paralysis, and 3% perforation [22] .There were no deaths. Another study by Cook et al. evaluating 74 endoscopic stapler-assisted diverticulotomies in 68 patients showed a total complication rate of 14%, including 7% dental injury, 4% postoperative fever, 1% transient vocal fold paralysis, and 1% perforation [25]. Similar complication rates were reported in Chang et al.'s study of 159 cases, with a total complication rate of 13%, including 7% dental injury, 4% postoperative fever, 1% aspiration pneumonia, 1% esophageal perforation, and 1% transient vocal fold paralysis [7].

Major complications commonly involve additional procedures and additional time in the hospital.

Management begins with prevention. The above discussion tries to convey information on how to perform the procedure safely. When complications do occur, they need to be dealt with expeditiously to minimize more serious outcomes.

Table 6.1 Potential complications of endoscopic staple diverticulostomy

Major complications	Minor complications
Pharyngeal perforation	Dental injury
Esophageal perforation	Pharyngeal laceration
Mediastinitis	Postoperative fever
Staple failure	Transient vocal fold paralysis
Aspiration pneumonia	

Management of Complications

Pharyngeal laceration is the most potentially serious complication and can be caused during placement of the laryngoscope or diverticuloscope, or, more commonly, placement of the stapler. This appears to occur in experienced hands in less than 3% of patients [8]. Laceration of the pharynx can happen with excessive pressure from the stapler in trying to engage the common wall of the pouch. The cartridge of the stapler is blunter, and it is another reason for introducing the stapler in the orientation of having the anvil in the diverticulum and the cartridge in the esophagus. If a laceration has occurred, it may well be possible to repair it endoscopically if it can be visualized [26] (Fig. 6.9). This repair usually occurs while the scope remains in

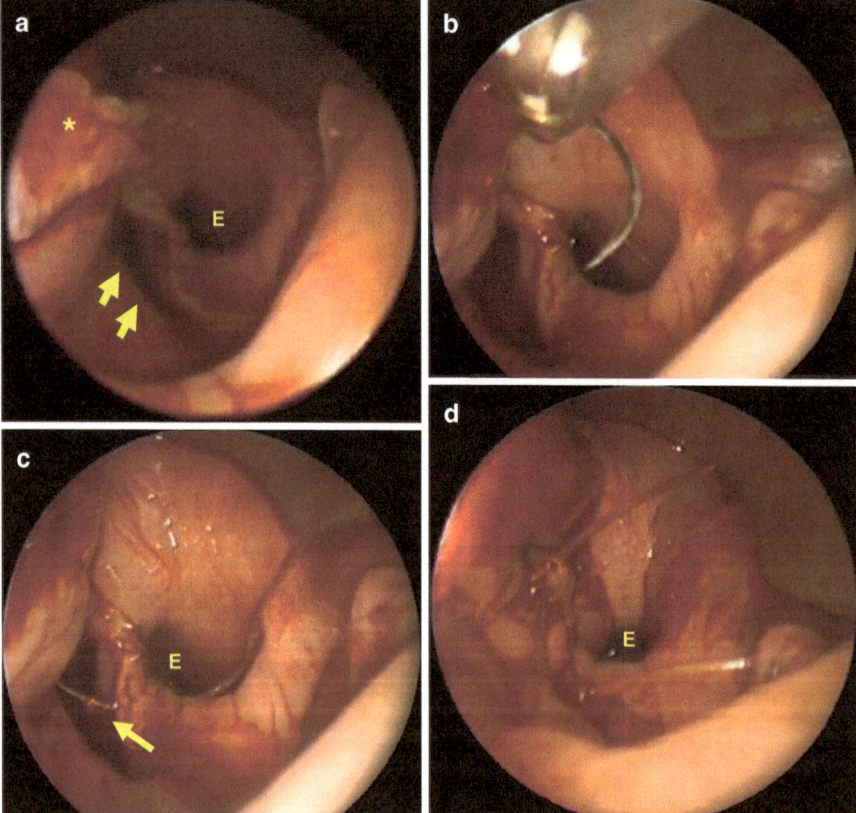

Fig. 6.9 Repair of a large mucosal laceration caused by the stapler anvil during ESD. Repair with endoscopic needle holder and surgical suture. (**a**) The laceration (arrows) is noted in the base of the ZD after creation of the esophagodiverticulostomy. Left edge of incision with staple closure is seen (asterisk). (**b**) The first suture needle is placed in the medial edge of the laceration. (**c**) The first suture is in place on one side of the laceration (arrow). (**d**) The knots are tied with a knot pusher and used as a retractor to place the subsequent sutures. Laceration closed primarily. Esophageal lumen (E)

suspension. Trying to replace the scope to properly visualize an injured segment may be very difficult.

In attempting to repair the laceration, the authors have found that the laparoscopic needle driver typically used by gastrointestinal surgeons is stronger and holds the needle better than the very fine "laryngeal" forceps promoted for laryngologists. It has curved jaws and holds the needle at a 45 degree angle. This allows suturing perpendicular to the plane of the shank of the needle driver similar to a Haney needle driver commonly used in gynecologic surgery. The needle is loaded on the outside of the curve, facing up. Telescopic visualization is used, and the needle driver is controlled with one hand. It can be very useful to have a foreign body-type alligator forceps with a toothed jaw for holding onto the mucosal laceration edges during the initial placement of sutures. Since the Endo Stitch never let go of the needle, another strategy is to place one stitch through any end of the laceration with this device and use it as a traction suture. A clamp attached to the ends of the suture providing light gravitational pull can help to stabilize tissue when suturing. Another similar technique is to place an initial suture (by any means) and leave that suture uncut to act as a retractor for the placement of any additional required sutures. The authors have used simple sutures to close such wounds, as trying to use mattress sutures leaves the doubled-over suture material in the barrel of the laryngoscope making placement of the second needle pass overly difficult. In general, it is a good idea to practice endoscopic repair prior to any clinical need and know what suture and needle driver is preferable.

If a laceration were to occur, it is considered advisable to place a nasogastric tube. The patient may have an extended recovery, and nutrition is important in this patient group. This should be performed endoscopically to ensure that the tube does not pass through the laceration into the mediastinum. Larger nasogastric tubes, especially those with Salem sump design, will not fit through all common endoscopes. Since most scopes are passed transorally and nasogastric by definition are passed transnasally, the end of the gastric tube must be picked up, visualizing it through the laryngoscope or esophagoscope, and pushed ahead of the scope. Other options are postoperative, radiologic placement of an NG tube or an endoscopic or laparoscopic PEG placement.

Stapler Line Leaks

Early detection of salivary leaks from non-visualized staple-line dehiscence or endoscopically repaired pharyngeal lacerations is critical in the management of this complication in order to try to prevent progression to mediastinitis. Patients who develop a leak typically complain of a mid-thoracic (intra-scapular) back pain, which is not typical of a postoperative discomfort from neck hyperextension or lumbar discomfort from lying flat on the operating table. It typically occurs very early in the postoperative period. Neck tenderness on examination and crepitus will be present in the case of large perforations and should be managed with immediate return to the operating room for direct neck exploration, repair (if possible), and drainage of the retropharyngeal space. Neck pain and tenderness should be addressed with a neck CT to look for free air. Waiting for temperature elevation or palpation of crepitus is not required to initiate a neck exploration and placement of a drain. Early treatment is usually successful in controlling mediastinitis, but an actual fistula may take longer to close. Even a laceration that is repaired transcervically should be drained, since the neck is already opened and a drain is easily removed if not needed.

Other Complications

Injury to the teeth and gums from laryngoscope pressure is certainly possible and well recognized for all rigid laryngoscopy procedures. Prevention is the best management, but when dental injury does occur, prompt consultation by dentistry is required. Pressure on the back of the larynx from the laryngoscope can lead to pressure on the recurrent laryngeal nerve giving the patient a temporary vocal cord paralysis. Vocal cord paralysis has been an extremely rare event after ESD and can be treated with vocal fold injection with absorbable material if the patient has a significant communication deficit or dysphagia.

Early postoperative dysphagia is usually the result of simple edema that will subside over a few days and can be managed with a thickened liquid diet. If one is confident that no leak has occurred and diabetes mellitus is not present, corticosteroids may hasten its resolution.

Patient-reported recurrence or persistence of dysphagia has been reported to occur in 7.1% of primary ESD patients, but diverticulum size was not significantly associated with failure [8]. This rate of symptom recurrence is similar to recurrence rates of 0% to 19% reported for external approaches with variable lengths of follow-up [7]. Recurrence may be a result of incomplete division of the cricopharyngeal muscle as well as restenosis of the common wall diverticulostomy from scarring. Findings of a partial or complete scar band at the earlier ESD diverticulostomy site for revision ESD support inflammatory factors in wound healing as an etiology, but definite causation has not been established.

Intraoperative measures to decrease the chance of recurrence include the use of retraction sutures to help position the common wall and allow the stapler to be placed for maximal sectioning. Removal of any loose staples or retained sutures immediately after the common wall is divided may help to prevent mucosal edge irritation and subsequent restenosis. ESD does not induce thermal injury and inflammation to the tissues, as do the CO_2 laser and electrocautery; this may help to limit scar tissue formation. Finally, control of medical factors other than ZD that may affect swallowing must be achieved to provide the greatest chance of symptom relief.

Patients who experience recurrence of ZD after primary excision by the transcervical route or by any manner of endoscopic diverticulostomy may undergo revision surgery with ESD. This has been shown to be effective, without any increase in technical difficulty or morbidity [27, 28]. However, revision ESD may not be the best option for those patients with a very small pouch (1 to 2 cm or less) who have had previous external diverticulectomy, because scarring from earlier treatment and small diverticular size make retraction of the common wall into the stapler blades difficult [28]. In this case, an external approach with cricopharyngeal myotomy may be more effective. However, external reoperations are technically demanding and have a much higher incidence of complication secondary to adhesions and distorted anatomy [29, 30].

Limitations

ESD does have its limitations, although they are few. As with all rigid transoral endoscopy, exposure of the diverticulum may be difficult or impossible because of patient anatomy, such as with kyphosis, large cervical osteophytes, or a small oropharyngeal opening. Small ZD (less than 2 cm) poses a technical challenge, as sufficient endoscopic division of the common wall is difficult given the dimensions of the stapler. Placement of retraction sutures improves the ability to engage the common wall in the stapler, so even a small pouch may be successfully treated. Even with these sutures, retraction of the common wall may not be possible in the patient with a recurrent small ZD from an earlier external approach because of scarring [28]. Collard and associates proposed that by sawing off the distal part of the Endo GIA 30 stapler anvil, a more complete section of the common wall to the bottom of the diverticulum could be accomplished [5]. However, in addition to its introducing avoidable risks to the procedure by potentially affecting the integrity of the staple closure, we have found such a modification unnecessary [6, 22].

Summary

ESD has been found to be a safe, effective, and efficient surgical intervention for treatment of Zenker diverticulum. Successful treatment is enhanced by knowledge of the instrumentation and its limitations. This is especially true of the endoscopic staplers. Awareness of potential complications and their treatment allows for better informed consent and management. The clinical results for ESD demonstrating excellent relief of dysphagia, rapid postoperative convalescence, and minimal morbidity support the use of this approach for the majority of patients with ZD.

References

1. Mosher HP. Webs and pouches of the esophagus, their diagnosis and treatment. Surg Gynecol Obstet. 1917;25:175–87.
2. Dohlman G, Mattsson L. The endoscopic operation for hypopharyngeal diverticula. A roent-gencinematographic study. Arch Otolaryngol Head Neck Surg. 1960;71:744–52.
3. van Overbeek JJ. Meditation on the pathogenesis of hypopharyngeal (Zenker's) diverticulum and a report of endoscopic treatment in 545 patients. Ann Otol Rhinol Laryngol. 1994;103:178–85.

4. Martin-Hirsch DP, Newbegin CJ. Autosuture GIA gun: a new application in the treatment of hypopharyngeal diverticula. J Laryngol Otol. 1993;107:723–5.
5. Collard JM, Otte JB, Kestens PJ. Endoscopic stapling technique of esophagodiverticulostomy for Zenker's diverticulum. Ann Thorac Surg. 1993;56:573–6.
6. Scher RL, Richtsmeier WJ. Endoscopic staple-assisted esophagodiverticulostomy for Zenker's diverticulum. Laryngoscope. 1996;106:951–6.
7. Chang C, Payyapilli R, Scher RL. Endoscopic staple diverticulostomy for Zenker's diverticulum: review of literature and experience in 159 consecutive patients. Laryngoscope. 2003;113:957–65.
8. Wilken R, Whited C, Scher RL. Endoscopic staple diverticulostomy for Zenker's diverticulum: review of experience in 337 cases. Ann Otol Rhinol Laryngol. 2015;124:21–9.
9. Thaler ER, Weber RS, Goldberg AN, Weinstein GS. Feasibility and outcome of endoscopic staple-assisted esophagodiverticulostomy for Zenker's diverticulum. Laryngoscope. 2001;111:1506–8.
10. Richtsmeier WJ. Myotomy length determinants in endoscopic staple-assisted esophagodiverticulostomy for small Zenker's diverticula. Ann Otol Rhinol Laryngol. 2005;114:341–6.
11. McGuire J, Wright IC, Leverment JN. Surgical staplers: a review. J R Coll Surg Edinb. 1997;42:1–9.
12. Richtsmeier WJ, Monzon JR. Postendoscopic Zenker esophagodiverticulostomy leaks associated with a specific stapler cartridge. Arch Otolaryngol Head Neck Surg. 2002;128:137–40.
13. Hollinger LD. Patient examination, endoscopy and biopsy. In: Cummings CW, Fredrickson JM, editors. Otolaryngology – head and neck surgery, vol. III. St. Louis: CV Mosby; 1986. p. 2264.
14. Acharya A, Jennings S, Douglas S, Mirza S, Beasley N. Carcinoma arising in a pharyngeal pouch previously treated by endoscopic stapling. Laryngoscope. 2006;116:1043–5.
15. Herbella FA, Dubecz A, Patti MG. Esophageal diverticula and cancer. Dis Esophagus. 2012;25:153–8.
16. Chekan E, Whelan RL. Surgical stapling device-tissue interactions: what surgeons need to know to improve patient outcomes. Med Devices (Auckl). 2014;7:305–18.
17. Roth JA, Sigston E, Vallance N. Endoscopic stapling of pharyngeal pouch: a 10-year review of single versus multiple staple rows. Otolaryngol Head Neck Surg. 2009;140:245–9.
18. Jaramillo MJ, McLay KA, McAteer D. Long-term clinico-radiological assessment of endoscopic stapling of pharyngeal pouch: a series of cases. J Laryngol Otol. 2001;115:462–6.
19. Ong CC, Elton PG, Mitchell D. Pharyngeal pouch endoscopic stapling—are post-operative barium swallow radiographs of any value? J Laryngol Otol. 1999;113:233–6.
20. Hadley JM, Ridley N, Djazaeri B, et al. The radiological appearances after the endoscopic cricopharyngeal myotomy: Dohlman's procedure. Clin Radiol. 1997;52:613–5.
21. Sydow B, Levine MS, Rubesin SE, et al. Radiographic findings and complications after surgical or endoscopic repair of Zenker's diverticulum in 16 patients. AJR Am J Roentgenol. 2001;177:1067–71.
22. Scher RL, Richtsmeier WJ. Long-term experience with endoscopic staple-assisted esophagodiverticulostomy for Zenker's diverticulum. Laryngoscope. 1998;108:200–5.
23. Peracchia A, Bonavina L, Narne S, et al. Minimally invasive surgery for Zenker's diverticulum: analysis of results in 95 consecutive patients. Arch Surg. 1998;133:695–700.
24. Barton MD, Detwiller KY, Palmer AD, Schindler JS. The safety and efficacy of endoscopic Zenker's diverticulotomy: a cohort study. Laryngoscope. 2016;126(12):2705–10.
25. Cook RD, Huang PC, Richstmeier WJ, et al. Endoscopic staple-assisted esophagodiverticulostomy: an excellent treatment of choice for Zenker's diverticulum. Laryngoscope. 2000;110:2020–5.
26. Paleri V, Najim O, Meikle D, Wilson JA. Microlaryngoscopic repair of iatrogenic pharyngeal pouch perforations: treatment of choice? Head Neck. 2007;29:189–92.
27. Koay CB, Commins D, Bates GJ. The role of endoscopic stapling diverticulotomy in recurrent pharyngeal pouch. J Laryngol Otol. 1998;112:954–5.

28. Scher RL. Endoscopic staple diverticulostomy for recurrent Zenker's diverticulum. Laryngoscope. 2003;113:63–7.
29. Payne WS. The treatment of pharyngoesophageal diverticulum: the simple and complex. Hepatogastroenterology. 1992;39:109–14.
30. Ellis F. Pharyngoesophageal (Zenker's) diverticulum. Adv Surg. 1995;28:171–89.

Non-staple Endoscopic Management of Zenker Diverticulum

Keith A. Chadwick, Joshua S. Schindler, and Natalie A. Krane

Introduction

The treatment of dysphagia associated with Zenker diverticula (ZD) has evolved since its description by Zenker and Ziemssen [1]. While initial attempts were made to manage these transorally, these efforts were largely abandoned because of limitations in exposure and concerns for patient safety. For many years through the early 1900s, surgeons approached Zenker diverticula through a transcervical approach in order to control the alimentary tract and drain expected fistulae. As recovery was protracted and complications such as fibrosis, fistula formation, and recurrent laryngeal nerve injury continued to occur, a less invasive—yet efficacious— method of surgical correction was sought through the latter half of the twentieth century. As a result of modifications in technique, equipment, and imaging, most surgeons now choose to manage ZD through endoscopic means, with open techniques reserved for ever fewer challenging cases.

Historical Considerations

Early attempts at diverticulotomy by an endoscopic approach were initiated in the early twentieth century. Jackson was the first to report his experience with esophagoscope-assisted diverticulectomy in 1915 [2]. This first attempt was a combined endoscopic and transcervical procedure, using a standard esophagoscope to remove retained debris from within the diverticulum, present and transilluminate the diverticulum through the external wound, and maintain the esophageal lumen during esophageal closure. Though the diverticulum was still excised in a

K. A. Chadwick · J. S. Schindler (✉) · N. A. Krane
Department of Otolaryngology—Head and Neck Surgery, Oregon Health and Science University, Portland, OR, USA
e-mail: schindlj@ohsu.edu

© Springer International Publishing AG, part of Springer Nature 2018
R. Scher, D. Myssiorek (eds.), *Management of Zenker and Hypopharyngeal Diverticula*, https://doi.org/10.1007/978-3-319-92156-3_7

transcervical fashion, this represented the first effort to use endoscopic techniques during diverticulectomy. Two years later, Mosher was the first to attempt an entirely endoscopic approach. During this procedure, the esophagoscope was used to visualize the diverticulum, and a surgical knife was used to cut the cricopharyngeal bar through the esophagoscope [3]. As visualization of the cricopharyngeal bar was limited during these procedures, the subsequent risk of mediastinitis was high. Indeed, the seventh patient that underwent this procedure developed mediastinitis and died. Thus, Mosher and other surgeons abandoned this technique in favor of transcervical approaches that could control leaks from the hypopharynx. Based on the high rate of morbidity and mortality seen in this limited experience in endoscopic management, open diverticulectomy remained the gold standard for the decades to follow. However, with advances in imaging, antibiotic therapy, optics, diverticuloscopes, and endoscopic tools, surgeons continued to seek safe and efficacious endoscopic approaches to treat ZD.

The first of these advances came in the form of exposure. By the late 1950s, Dohlman developed a modified esophagoscope, which displayed two "lips" (one placed into the esophagus and one placed into the diverticulum) allowing for exposure of the common diverticular and esophageal wall and the ability to place it on tension for more controlled surgical division. By utilizing this modified esophagoscope, diathermic coagulation (similar in many ways to monopolar electrocautery) could be utilized to divide the cricopharyngeus [4]. In Dohlman's experience of nearly 100 cases, there were no cases of severe complications (including death or mediastinitis), and a recurrence rate of 7% was reported. This published experience gave more surgeons the confidence that endoscopic diverticulotomy could be safe and efficacious and laid the foundation for further development and experimentation.

With improved exposure of the cricopharyngeal bar, further modifications to Dohlman's technique sought to allow even more controlled division of the cricopharyngeal muscle and overlying mucosa with the operating microscope [5] and surgical lasers (both carbon dioxide [5] and potassium titanyl phosphate [6]). While technically feasible and likely superior to electrosurgical endoscopic approaches, the use of the surgical microscope and laser was not commonly available and still required a great deal of skill. Surgeons continued to seek a simpler solution to the problem of controlled cricopharyngeal bar division. The answer came in 1993, when both Collard and Martin-Hirsch independently published reports of performing a stapled diverticulotomy with an endoscopic gastrointestinal anastomosis stapler (Multifire Endo GIA 30, Medtronic, Minneapolis, MN) [7, 8]. Both reports demonstrated the safety of these instruments when applied to ZD, and surgeons rapidly embraced this technique. By the mid-1990s, endoscopic stapler-assisted diverticulotomy became the procedure of choice by most surgeons for the treatment of ZD.

The widespread application of the endoscopic stapler was made possible through contemporaneous refinements to Dohlman's original modified esophagoscope. Further evolution occurred with the development of the Weerda diverticuloscope (Karl Storz Endoscopy, Tuttlingen, Germany). Developed in Germany, this was the

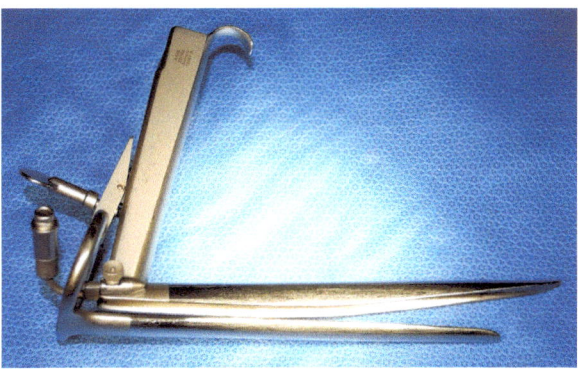

Fig. 7.1 The Weerda diverticuloscope (Karl Storz Endoscopy, Tuttlingen, Germany). For reference, see Lang et al. [45]

first scope to utilize a bivalved design, in which both the proximal and distal openings could be widened or collapsed (Fig. 7.1). This esophagoscope design provided markedly improved visualization of the common wall. This visualization was essential for application of the endoscopic stapler in many cases and allowed the diverticulum wall to be placed under greater tension for division with a laser.

Despite the simplicity of the laparoscopic stapler to perform diverticulotomy and cricopharyngeal myotomy and its widespread application, surgeons recognized that this treatment was not universally effective. Difficulties in exposure and the presence of small diverticula that did not allow complete division of the cricopharyngeus muscle limited the use of the endoscopic stapler to a subset of intermediate-sized diverticula that could be suitably exposed for the 12-mm-diameter stapler. While some surgeons continued to use carbon dioxide lasers to address these smaller lesions, others sought innovative solutions to this problem. Scher and his colleagues used a laparoscopic suture applier to encircle the cricopharyngeus muscle on either side of the diverticulotomy [9]. Traction could be applied to these sutures to pull the cricopharyngeus muscle into the stapler for more complete division. Other innovative endoscopic techniques in the twenty-first century have been reported, including the use of ultrasonic high-frequency transduction (Harmonic scalpel, Ethicon Inc., Somerville, NJ) [10] or bipolar diathermy (LigaSure, Medtronic, Minneapolis, MN) [11]. The Harmonic scalpel was felt to "seal" the diverticulum mucosa and submucosa thus providing a safer means to divide smaller diverticula than the carbon dioxide laser. While reports of this technique are limited to relatively small cohorts of patients, the most recent evaluation of this approach suggests an unacceptably high complication rate to merit widespread application [12].

Outcomes for treatment of ZD via transoral means remain excellent with high first-treatment success and low complication rates. A large retrospective study by van Overbeek et al. of 545 patients treated endoscopically by a variety of techniques (including diathermic electrocoagulation and carbon dioxide laser) showed that 91% of patients reported "high satisfaction" with the procedure [13]. A large meta-review published in 2004 shows a satisfactory outcome in 96% of patients treated endoscopically, with a 6% persistence/recurrence rate and a 3% rate of major morbidity (including a 2.6% rate of esophageal perforation or leak) [14]. A recent retrospective review by Barton of 106 consecutive patients undergoing either laser-assisted or stapler-assisted endoscopic Zenker diverticulotomy demonstrated an overall satisfaction rating of 8.2 on a 10-point scale with no major complications [15].

Modern Endoscopic Approaches

Modern endoscopic techniques for safe and successful management of ZD require careful consideration of patient factors. Successful intervention mandates adequate exposure of the diverticulum and esophagodiverticular, or "party," wall containing the cricopharyngeus muscle. Once exposed, a variety of techniques can be used to intervene upon the diverticulum in an effective manner. Following the procedure, cautious advancement of oral intake may be initiated, or imaging should be obtained to ensure the absence of an esophageal leak or perforation.

Preoperative Considerations

A comprehensive preoperative work-up is imperative for appropriate patient selection prior to endoscopic procedures for ZD. All patients should undergo radiographic imaging with either an esophagram or modified barium swallow study (MBSS) to evaluate the size and location of the pouch. MBSS with esophageal follow-through, a functional study, is the preferred imaging modality, which allows for assessment of comorbid pharyngoesophageal conditions. Diverticula that are longer than 2 cm and adequate to expose may be considered for stapler-assisted ZD, while others may be treated with the laser [15]. Furthermore, an assessment of anatomic factors that may limit exposure of the diverticulum from an endoscopic approach should be pursued. Patients who may be at risk for unsuccessful endoscopic exposure of the diverticular sac include those with small ZD (<2 cm), retrognathic mandibles, large tongues, kyphosis, or decreased neck mobility [16].

Exposure

Rigid diverticuloscopy is performed under general anesthesia with neuromuscular blockade. Once general anesthesia is obtained and the patient is intubated, the patient is typically rotated 90° or 180° away from the anesthesia team. The patient is then placed into the "sniffing position," with extension of the neck and slight flexion of the atlanto-occipital joint. The dentition or maxilla is protected in all cases with either a durable pre-molded dental guard or thermoplastic sheeting (Aquaplast, Allied Medical Products, Tarzana, CA) molded to the patient's dentition. Such protection is essential as the forces on the maxillary dentition can be substantial during rigid diverticuloscopy. Unlike direct laryngoscopy, the surgeon should also be careful to observe the mandibular dentition during exposure and suspension, as the distending diverticuloscopes can apply pressure to these teeth in many cases. If the patient is edentulous, a moist gauze may be used to protect the maxillary mucosa.

Rigid exposure for direct transoral endoscopic intervention is performed using a diverticuloscope to expose the cricopharyngeus (CP) muscle. As previously stated, the Weerda endoscope is preferred once the patient is correctly positioned, and the diverticuloscope is then placed gently into the oral cavity and advanced past the base of the tongue and epiglottis and through the oropharynx to the postcricoid hypopharynx. It is important to remember to insert and advance the scope with the distal and proximal openings in a collapsed or closed position. Surgical lubricant may facilitate advancing the scope and minimize mucosal injury. The scope is then advanced until the flanges of the scope expose the CP muscle, with the posterior flange proximal to the diverticulum and the anterior flange proximal to the esophagus. When using an articulating diverticuloscope, the proximal and distal openings are then widened to place the diverticuloesophageal wall containing the cricopharyngeus muscle wall on stretch. The diverticuloscope is then suspended using a suspension arm (Karl Storz Endoscopy, Tuttlingen, Germany) and a mustard table (Medtronic, Dublin, Ireland), allowing for adequate visualization of the CP muscle (Fig. 7.2) [15, 17]. At this point, correct placement of the diverticuloscope may be confirmed by using a nasogastric tube or bougie stylet to palpate the diverticular pouch and esophagus.

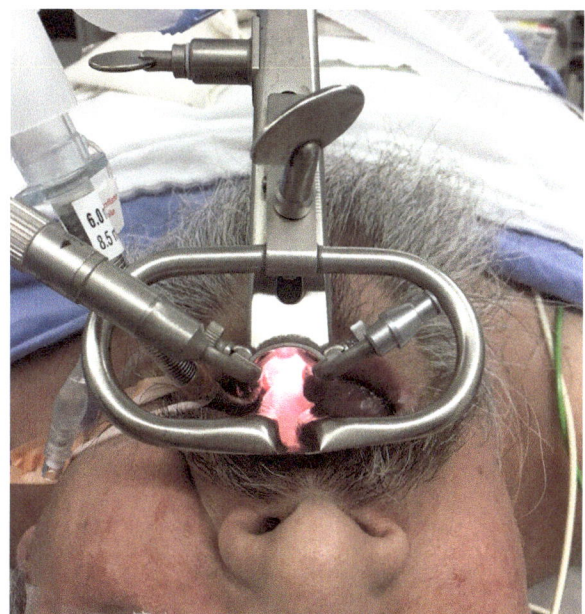

Fig. 7.2 The Weerda diverticuloscope in use for transoral exposure of a Zenker diverticulum

If entry into the cervical esophagus is challenging because of hypertonicity or fibrosis of the cricopharyngeus muscle, careful dilation of the esophagus may be performed. This can be performed under direct visualization either with the use of Savary-Gilliard dilators (over a guidewire), serial dilations of the upper esophageal sphincter from 21 to 42 Fr [20], or a controlled radial expansion (CRE) balloon catheter [17]. The authors prefer to pass a bougie into the cervical esophageal introitus and follow this with the anterior flange of the diverticuloscope. This is effective in almost all cases and does not cause significant trauma in our experience.

Once adequate exposure of the diverticular wall is achieved, the diverticulopharyngeal wall can then be divided by a variety of techniques. Endoscopic staplers, laser, cold instruments, bipolar diathermy, and harmonic scalpel have all been used recently for this technique. The endoscopic staple approach will be covered in a separate chapter.

Laser-Assisted Diverticulotomy

Endoscopic stapler-assisted Zenker diverticulotomy may not be adequately or easily performed secondary to small pouch size or patient anatomical factors resulting in limited exposure. In these cases, an endoscopic laser-assisted diverticulotomy should be considered. In general, laser techniques can be performed on diverticula smaller than 2 cm since the laser is able to divide the diverticulopharyngeal wall more completely than the stapler [18]. Additionally, endoscopic laser diverticulotomy may require less exposure when compared to endoscopic stapler-assisted procedures and may allow the endoscopic procedure to be completed in cases which previously would have been aborted [15]. Historically, endoscopic laser cricopharyngeal myotomy has been performed using both the potassium-titanyl-phosphate (KTP) laser [6, 19] and carbon dioxide (CO_2) laser [5]. The CO_2 laser is likely superior for this procedure as it is easier to control on a micromanipulator attached to the microscope and better at cutting tissue with less thermal artifact and char than the KTP laser.

Technique

As with any procedure involving laser use, a laser safety checklist should be performed prior to using a laser device, ensuring the use of eye protection by the patient and staff and determining that laser settings are correct and the laser has been test fired, irrigation is available on the surgical field, and all staff are aware of fire extinguisher locations. Following adequate exposure of the ZD wall, a CO_2 or KTP laser is then used with a micromanipulator attached to the operating microscope to divide the CP muscle until the muscular fibers are completely transected and the diverticular pouch is flushed with the esophagus [17] (Figs. 7.3 and 7.4). Cervical esophageal fibers that contribute to the upper esophageal sphincter can also be divided for 5–10 mm inferiorly just under the esophageal submucosa. The laser should be used to cautiously divide all of the cricopharyngeal muscle fibers layer by layer to ensure a complete myotomy without inadvertent injury to the buccopharyngeal fascia that invests the entire pharyngoesophageal segment. Hemostasis is generally easy to achieve with the laser and topical 1:10,000 epinephrine on cotton pledgets. In rare cases, more troublesome bleeding may be treated with judicious monopolar cautery,

Fig. 7.3 Transoral use of the CO_2 laser to divide the mucosa. Note the well-defined cricopharyngeus muscle fibers within the diverticulopharyngeal party wall

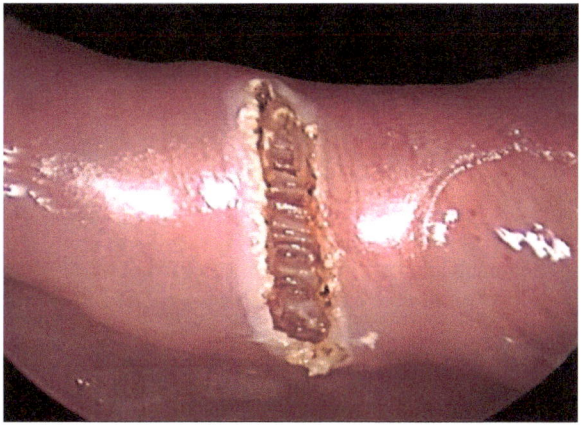

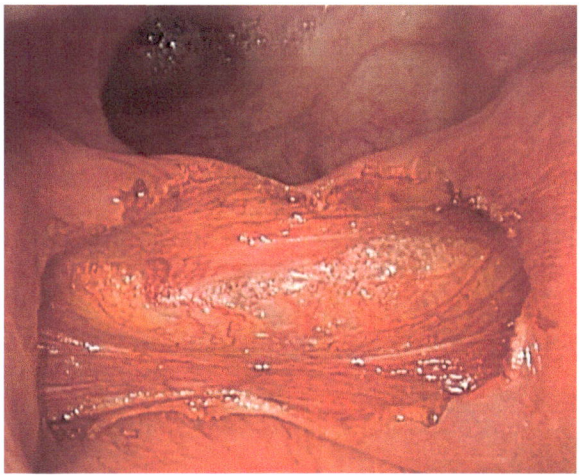

Fig. 7.4 Demonstration of the buccopharyngeal fascia and cervical esophagus within the diverticulopharyngeal party wall after the use of the CO_2 laser for diverticulotomy and cricopharyngeal myotomy. This fascia prevents leakage from the alimentary tract into the prevertebral space. Note that the cricopharyngeus muscle is completely divided and retracts laterally deep under the mucosa when under tension

thrombin, or microfibrillar collagen hemostat application (Avitene, Davol, subsidiary of CR Bard, Warwick, RI). A laser-shielded or metal endotracheal tube should be used and communication with the anesthesiologist that a laser is about to be used should be undertaken to assure that the end tidal oxygen level is brought to its lowest allowable concentration. The authors prefer to use room air for ventilation whenever possible to minimize the risk of a laser airway fire.

Careful attention and operator experience are required to safely complete the myotomy without creating an esophageal perforation. The myotomy should only be performed when the CP muscle can be adequately visualized, and dissection should stop once the deepest muscle fiber is divided and the buccopharyngeal fascia is visualized. Aside from utilizing extreme caution, several techniques have been described to prevent esophageal perforation. Primary mucosal closure with Vicryl suture has been described [20]. Alternatively, some authors recommend avoiding division of the soft tissue all the way down to the buccopharyngeal fascia and instead use a CRE balloon to dilate the cricopharyngeal area to 18–20 mm after a laser-assisted partial myotomy is performed [17]. These techniques are not routinely performed—nor are they required in the authors' opinion—and their usage largely depends on the operator's preference and comfort level.

Outcomes
Patients undergoing endoscopic laser treatment of ZD report overall satisfaction with the procedure. In an early series of ten patients treated with KTP laser diverticulotomy, all were either "very satisfied" or "satisfied" with their results, and none of the patients required further treatment after diverticulotomy [6]. Four of these patients had evidence of a residual pouch on postoperative MBSS, of which two patients experienced mild persistent pill dysphagia. In a study of 37 patients undergoing laser-assisted diverticulotomy, a 92% long-term satisfaction rate was noted, with 70% complete resolution and 22% partial resolution of symptoms [21]. A large patient satisfaction study, evaluating 507 patients treated endoscopically with carbon dioxide laser-assisted myotomy (with or without diathermy for hemostasis) showed a 99% satisfaction rate [22]. Additionally, the majority of patients experience a significant reduction in their symptoms, including a subjective reduction in dysphagia and regurgitation in 91% [23], reduction in functional outcome swallowing scale (FOSS) scores by 1.4 of 6 points [17], and significant reduction in EAT-10 scores by 11.2 points [15]. These improvements seemed durable in the vast majority of these patients with an average follow-up of over 4 years.

Complications
Potential complications of endoscopic laser-assisted diverticulotomy are similar to that of stapler-assisted procedures and include esophageal perforation, which may require external drainage, mediastinitis, dental injury, subcutaneous emphysema, bleeding, temporary regurgitation of liquids, and throat pain [15, 24]. In the aforementioned patient satisfaction study, an 8% complication rate was identified, including 2% rate of mediastinitis [22]. In Kuhn's series evaluating KTP laser diverticulotomy of ten patients, 10% had subcutaneous emphysema, and 20% had postoperative fever (over 101.5 °F), though there were no major complications [6].

Endoscopic Stapler-Assisted Versus Laser-Assisted Diverticulotomy

Both stapler-assisted and laser-assisted techniques can be successfully used to manage patients with ZD and provide myriad benefits over the traditional open approach. Endoscopic techniques lead to similar or better outcomes and have fewer complications. When compared to an open approach, laser techniques offer an improved postoperative course, shorter operative time, and potentially shorter hospital course [25]. Stapler-assisted techniques offer shorter operative time, reduced hospital stay, earlier initiation of oral intake, and lower overall complication rates [26–32].

Outcomes

Both endoscopic laser-assisted and stapler-assisted Zenker diverticulotomy offer symptom relief and a high degree of patient satisfaction [21, 32]. Postoperative outcomes with regard to swallowing are similar despite method of endoscopic management. In the 2016 study by Barton et al., an improvement in postoperative dysphagia scores on the EAT-10 improved by an average of 8.0 points out of 40, with no statistically significant difference in improvement based on endoscopic technique [15]. It is important to note that this study was not a head-to-head comparison of techniques, rather an analysis of safety and efficacy of endoscopic treatment using both stapler- and laser-assisted techniques to resolve symptoms by transoral means. Secondary outcomes, such as length of hospitalization or length of time to initiation of oral intake, can be difficult to compare between the two techniques since most centers use different postoperative protocols for each procedure. Regardless, Chang et al. performed a review of the literature as it pertains to the endoscopic surgical treatment for ZD and found that those treated with laser-assisted diverticulotomy experience an average of 2.2 days to initiation of oral intake and mean hospital stay of 6.5 days, compared to an average of 1.0 day to initiation of oral intake and a mean hospital stay of 1.8 days in the stapler-assisted group [25]. Therefore, postoperative outcomes favoring stapler-assisted technique include a shorter duration of *nil per os* (NPO) status [26, 40] and a decreased length of hospitalization [16, 18, 33]. Additionally, a lower incidence of postoperative fevers [18] and abnormal chest X-rays are seen following stapler-assisted Zenker diverticulotomy [33]. On the contrary, though patients undergoing either laser- and stapler-assisted endoscopic diverticulotomy experience significant improvement in both dysphagia and regurgitation [15, 16, 34], a greater improvement in these outcomes has been shown in those patients who underwent laser-assisted procedures in some studies [15, 33, 34].

Revision Rate

In most studies, a lower revision rate has been reported in those undergoing endoscopic laser Zenker diverticulotomy as compared to endoscopic staple-assisted diverticulotomy [33–35]. Other reports have demonstrated no significant difference in revision rate when comparing endoscopic stapler-assisted and laser-assisted techniques [15, 18, 33]. If reoperation is required, however, the length of time to reoperation has been shown to be significantly shorter in the stapler-assisted group [18]. Because a more complete and precise diverticulotomy can be performed with the laser, this may contribute to the lower revision rate seen compared to stapler-assisted procedures [15, 34].

Complications

Complications in both procedures are typically uncommon and relatively minor, and mortality after both procedures has rarely been reported [34, 35]. The most common operative complication of either endoscopic technique was dental trauma [34], which may be prevented by the judicious use of dental protection and careful insertion and suspension of the diverticuloscope. An increased risk of non-dental complications is seen with the CO_2 laser technique; however, no statistically significant difference in overall complications, dental complications, or major complications is reported in most studies [33]. The Barton et al. study demonstrated an overall complication rate of 8% when evaluating all methods of endoscopic diverticulotomy, though all of the complications were noted in patients undergoing a laser-assisted procedure [15]. All complications were minor, including transient subcutaneous emphysema (5%), dental injury (2%), esophageal perforation (1%), and temporary regurgitation of liquids (1%). In Chang et al.'s literature review, patients undergoing endoscopic laser-assisted Zenker diverticulotomy experienced a complication rate of 7.4%, compared to a complication rate of 2.6% in stapler-assisted diverticulotomy [26]. Other studies have shown overall higher complication rates: 31% in laser procedures and 11% in stapler-assisted procedures [16]. Cervical subcutaneous emphysema or the presence of extra-esophageal air on lateral neck X-ray has been reported to occur more frequently in those patients undergoing laser diverticulotomy. When this occurs, it frequently resolves within 24 h without further complication (such as radiographic evidence of perforation) but must be followed until resolution [16, 18, 34].

Alternative Methods of Endoscopic Diverticulotomy

In recent decades, additional methods of endoscopic diverticulotomy have been explored. These techniques utilize alternative means for dividing the tissue within the common wall and performing the cricopharyngeal myotomy.

In 2009, Fama et al. was the first to describe the use of the Harmonic scalpel to perform the endoscopic diverticulotomy [10]. The Harmonic scalpel (Ethicon Inc., Somerville, NJ) is an ultrasonic transduction device, by which high-frequency vibrations in the transducer tip, creating mechanical energy, divide and coagulate tissue. This high-frequency disruption of tissues results in low-temperature coagulation and is commonly utilized in other head and neck procedures, including neck dissection and thyroidectomy. In this initial report, 25 patients were treated with the Harmonic scalpel, and complication rates were similar to other endoscopic techniques (8% postoperative chest pain, 4% postoperative cardiac event, 4% aspiration pneumonia, 4% transient cervical emphysema). Several additional smaller case series [36–38] showed similar rates of persistent symptoms and complications when comparing Harmonic scalpel-assisted and traditional endoscopic techniques. One study even reported the safe and efficacious use of a Harmonic scalpel through a flexible endoscope [39]. However, a more recent and larger series showed an increased rate of complications in Harmonic scalpel-assisted procedures (25%) compared to stapler-assisted procedures (5%) [12].

Another method recently introduced in the literature is endoscopic diverticulotomy with bipolar diathermic electrocoagulation (LigaSure, Medtronic, Minneapolis, MN) [11]. This electrosurgical device uses bipolar cautery to effect rapid coagulation and division of tissue. While similar to ultrasonic electrosurgery, this method may create similar tissue coagulum with less thermal injury and reduce the risk of fibrosis and stenosis at the surgical site. First described by Nielsen et al. in 2010 for the treatment of ZD in 15 patients, 80% of patients treated with bipolar electrocautery had resolution of symptoms in the long term, although 1 patient (7%) had an esophageal perforation requiring treatment with long-term antibiotics [11]. Several small case studies show promising efficacy and complication rates, which are similar to standard endoscopic techniques [40–43]. However, given the lack of large patient studies with long-term results, further study is needed to determine whether these alternative methods may replace more widely accepted techniques.

Postoperative Management

The management of patients undergoing endoscopic Zenker diverticulotomy in the immediate postoperative period is crucial to a safe and efficacious outcome. Although postoperative management protocols differ based on institution and surgeon preference, general guidelines and principles should be followed. Management also differs by type of endoscopic procedure performed. For example, since endoscopic laser diverticulotomy places patients at higher risk for esophageal perforation, they should be observed more closely or kept NPO longer than those undergoing a stapler-assisted procedure. The focus of postoperative management should be to reduce the risk of mediastinitis and infection. Signs and symptoms of mediastinitis include tachycardia, fever, chest pain, EKG changes, diaphoresis, and a general sense of unexplained discomfort and require immediate evaluation and intervention.

Postoperative management protocols following endoscopic cricopharyngeal myotomy vary in the literature and among practitioners, without a standard algorithm or process by which to follow. One published protocol immediately advances patients to a clear liquid diet on postoperative day 0 and to a soft diet on postoperative day 1 with discharge once diet is tolerated [17]. Another protocol maintains NPO until postoperative day 1, at which time they are initiated on a clear liquid diet and advanced to a soft mechanical diet prior to discharge home [16]. In a more conservative approach, patients are kept NPO until postoperative day 3, when they are advanced to a clear liquid diet and then to a full liquid diet prior to discharge, with advancement to a mechanical soft and regular diet as an outpatient [34].

In general, patients undergoing stapler-assisted endoscopic diverticulotomy are at lowest risk for esophageal perforation; this is due to the staple lines sealing the mucosal incisions along the diverticulopharyngeal wall and creating a water-tight seal of the tissue edges. Therefore, the postoperative management protocol tends to be more liberal than with other procedures. In the absence of concerning symptoms or findings in recovery, patients may be discharged home the same day and initiate a clear liquid diet on postoperative day 0. Indeed, a study by Gross et al. demonstrated the safety of discharge home from the recovery room on a liquid and soft food diet in uncomplicated cases if the patients could swallow adequately before discharge [44]. It is important to note that patients should be counseled extensively regarding symptoms concerning for mediastinitis and advised to present immediately to an emergency department should they develop concern for these. If the patient tolerates the clear liquid diet, they may be advanced to a soft mechanical diet and maintained on this until they are seen in follow-up several weeks later.

Patients undergoing laser-assisted endoscopic diverticulotomy are likely safest if observed until at least postoperative day 1. As the mucosal incisions are not routinely closed in these procedures, the risk for esophageal perforation is significant. Overnight observation allows the patient to be monitored for signs of mediastinitis, allowing for prompt diagnosis and management. Subcutaneous emphysema may be seen occasionally and, although worrisome, does not necessarily herald the development of mediastinitis. Though not all practitioners will obtain routine postoperative imaging, an esophagram obtained prior to initiation of oral intake can rule out a significant esophageal perforation. The absence of concerning findings on imaging can allow the practitioner to feel confident initiating oral intake trials if there is no evidence of leak [15, 18]. The patient is then advanced to a diet of all liquids and soft foods and discharged home. In our experience, patients may advance their own diet after 2 weeks to an unrestricted diet and be seen at approximately 4 weeks to assess response to surgery.

Some authors do not advocate for routine standard imaging unless there is clinical concern postoperatively. In those patients who demonstrate clinical concern for a postoperative complication, a lateral neck X-ray or CT neck and chest should be considered. If this demonstrates free air within the neck, the patient should be maintained NPO, and serial daily imaging examinations should be obtained until resolution is evident. If clinical decompensation or failure of resolution is apparent, a radiographic swallow study should be obtained to assess for a leak [17]. If at any point an esophageal perforation is identified, a nasogastric feeding tube should be placed under fluoroscopic guidance, and the patient maintained NPO for at least 1 week. Such placement may be challenging, and, as such, the authors (and others) choose to place a 10–12 Fr. nasogastric tube in all patients who undergo laser-assisted diverticulotomy or have anything to suggest concern during stapler-assisted diverticulotomy [15, 18].

The algorithms for postoperative diet advancement described above are not necessarily applicable to patients who were fed preoperatively via a gastrostomy tube or are at high risk of aspiration; instead, these patients require additional assessment and consideration prior to initiation of an oral diet.

Conclusion

ZD can be safely and effectively managed with endoscopic techniques. Through technological and procedural advancements, the vast majority of patients can be treated endoscopically. Patients with large ZD and favorable anatomy should be treated with stapler-assisted endoscopic diverticulotomy. However, patients with more difficult diverticular exposure, recurrent diverticula, or smaller diverticula may require a laser-assisted endoscopic approach. Although these approaches are preferred, other minimally invasive techniques, such as septotomy via flexible esophagoscopy, remain available as alternatives. With careful patient selection, precise surgical technique, and conservative postoperative practices, patients with ZD treated endoscopically have minimal risk of complications and excellent functional results.

References

1. Zenker FA, Zeimssen H. Dilatations of the esophagus. Cyclopedia Pract Med. 1878;3:46–8.
2. Gaub OJ, Jackson C. Pulsion diverticulum of the esophagus: a new operation for its cure. Surg Gynecol Obstet. 1915;21:52.
3. Mosher HP. Webs and pouches of the oesophagus, their diagnosis and treatment. Surg Gynecol Obstet. 1917;25:175–87.
4. Dohlman G, Mattsson O. The endoscopic operation for hypopharyngeal diverticula: a roentgencinematographic study. AMA Arch Otolaryngol. 1960;71:744–52.
5. van Overbeek JJ, Hoeksema PE, Edens ET. Microendoscopic surgery of the hypopharyngeal diverticulum using electrocoagulation or carbon dioxide laser. Ann Otol Rhinol Laryngol. 1984;93(1 Pt 1):34–6.
6. Kuhn FA, Bent JP III. Zenker's diverticulotomy using the KTP/532 laser. Laryngoscope. 1992;102(8):946–50.
7. Collard JM, Otte JB, Kestens PJ. Endoscopic stapling technique of esophagodiverticulostomy for Zenker's diverticulum. Ann Thorac Surg. 1993;56(3):573–6.
8. Martin-Hirsch DP, Newbegin CJ. Autosuture GIA gun: a new application in the treatment of hypopharyngeal diverticula. J Laryngol Otol. 1993;107(8):723–5.
9. Scher RL, Richtsmeier WJ. Endoscopic staple-assisted esophagodiverticulostomy for Zenker's diverticulum. Laryngoscope. 1996;106(8):951–6.
10. Fama AF, Moore EJ, Kasperbauer JL. Harmonic scalpel in the treatment of Zenker's diverticulum. Laryngoscope. 2009;119(7):1265–9.
11. Nielsen HU, Trolle W, Rubek N, Homoe P. New technique using LigaSure for endoscopic mucomyotomy of Zenker's diverticulum: diverticulotomy made easier. Laryngoscope. 2014;124(9):2039–42.
12. Whited C, Lee WT, Scher R. Evaluation of endoscopic harmonic diverticulostomy. Laryngoscope. 2012;122(6):1297–300.
13. van Overbeek JJ. Meditation on the pathogenesis of hypopharyngeal (Zenker's) diverticulum and a report of endoscopic treatment in 545 patients. Ann Otol Rhinol Laryngol. 1994;103(3):178–85.
14. Aly A, Devitt PG, Jamieson GG. Evolution of surgical treatment for pharyngeal pouch. Br J Surg. 2004;91(6):657–64.
15. Barton MD, Detwiller KY, Palmer AD, Schindler JS. The safety and efficacy of endoscopic Zenker's diverticulotomy: a cohort study. Laryngoscope. 2016;126(12):2705–10.
16. Miller FR, Bartley J, Otto RA. The endoscopic management of Zenker diverticulum: CO2 laser versus endoscopic stapling. Laryngoscope. 2006;116(9):1608–11.
17. Bergeron JL, Chhetri DK. Indications and outcomes of endoscopic CO2 laser cricopharyngeal myotomy. Laryngoscope. 2014;124(4):950–4.
18. Verhaegen VJ, Feuth T, van den Hoogen FJ, Marres HA, Takes RP. Endoscopic carbon dioxide laser diverticulostomy versus endoscopic staple-assisted diverticulostomy to treat Zenker's diverticulum. Head Neck. 2011;33(2):154–9.

19. Halvorson DJ, Kuhn FA. Transmucosal cricopharyngeal myotomy with the potassium-titanyl-phosphate laser in the treatment of cricopharyngeal dysmotility. Ann Otol Rhinol Laryngol. 1994;103(3):173–7.
20. Ho AS, Morzaria S, Damrose EJ. Carbon dioxide laser-assisted endoscopic cricopharyngeal myotomy with primary mucosal closure. Ann Otol Rhinol Laryngol. 2011;120(1):33–9.
21. Nyrop M, Svendstrup F, Jorgensen KE. Endoscopic CO2 laser therapy of Zenker's diverticulum--experience from 61 patients. Acta Otolaryngol Suppl. 2000;543:232–4.
22. Wouters B, van Overbeek JJ. Endoscopic treatment of the hypopharyngeal (Zenker's) diverticulum. Hepatogastroenterology. 1992;39(2):105–8.
23. Anagiotos A, Feyka M, Eslick GD, Lichtenstein T, Henning TD, Guntinas-Lichius O, et al. Long-term symptom control after endoscopic laser-assisted diverticulotomy of Zenker's diverticulum. Auris Nasus Larynx. 2014;41(6):568–71.
24. Lim RY. Endoscopic CO2 laser cricopharyngeal myotomy. J Clin Laser Med Surg. 1995;13(4):241–7.
25. Chang CW, Burkey BB, Netterville JL, Courey MS, Garrett CG, Bayles SW. Carbon dioxide laser endoscopic diverticulotomy versus open diverticulectomy for Zenker's diverticulum. Laryngoscope. 2004;114(3):519–27.
26. Chang CY, Payyapilli RJ, Scher RL. Endoscopic staple diverticulostomy for Zenker's diverticulum: review of literature and experience in 159 consecutive cases. Laryngoscope. 2003;113(6):957–65.
27. Gutschow CA, Hamoir M, Rombaux P, Otte JB, Goncette L, Collard JM. Management of pharyngoesophageal (Zenker's) diverticulum: which technique? Ann Thorac Surg. 2002;74(5):1677–82, discussion 1682–3.
28. Philippsen LP, Weisberger EC, Whiteman TS, Schmidt JL. Endoscopic stapled diverticulotomy: treatment of choice for Zenker's diverticulum. Laryngoscope. 2000;110(8):1283–6.
29. Raut VV, Primrose WJ. Long-term results of endoscopic stapling diverticulotomy for pharyngeal pouches. Otolaryngol Head Neck Surg. 2002;127(3):225–9.
30. Scher RL. Endoscopic staple diverticulostomy for recurrent Zenker's diverticulum. Laryngoscope. 2003;113(1):63–7.
31. Smith SR, Genden EM, Urken ML. Endoscopic stapling technique for the treatment of Zenker diverticulum vs standard open-neck technique: a direct comparison and charge analysis. Arch Otolaryngol Neck Surg. 2002;128(2):141–4.
32. van Eeden S, Lloyd RV, Tranter RM. Comparison of the endoscopic stapling technique with more established procedures for pharyngeal pouches: results and patient satisfaction survey. J Laryngol Otol. 1999;113(3):237–40.
33. Parker NP, Misono S. Carbon dioxide laser versus stapler-assisted endoscopic Zenker's diverticulotomy: a systematic review and meta-analysis. Otolaryngol Head Neck Surg. 2014;150(5):750–3.
34. Adam SI, Paskhover B, Sasaki CT. Laser versus stapler: outcomes in endoscopic repair of Zenker diverticulum. Laryngoscope. 2012;122(9):1961–6.
35. Pollei TR, Hinni ML, Hayden RE, Lott DG, Mors MB. Comparison of carbon dioxide laser-assisted versus stapler-assisted endoscopic cricopharyngeal myotomy. Ann Otol Rhinol Laryngol. 2013;122(9):568–74.
36. Allen J, Belafsky PC. Endoscopic cricopharyngeal myotomy for Zenker diverticulum using the harmonic scalpel. Ear Nose Throat J. 2010;89(5):216–8.
37. May JT 4th, Padhya TA, McCaffrey TV. Endoscopic repair of Zenker's diverticulum by harmonic scalpel. Am J Otolaryngol. 2011;32(6):553–6.
38. Sharp DB, Newman JR, Magnuson JS. Endoscopic management of Zenker's diverticulum: stapler assisted versus Harmonic Ace. Laryngoscope. 2009;119(10):1906–12.
39. Hondo FY, Maluf-Filho F, Giordano-Nappi JH, Neves CZ, Cecconello I, Sakai P. Endoscopic treatment of Zenker's diverticulum by harmonic scalpel. Gastrointest Endosc. 2011;74(3):666–71.
40. Andersen MF, Trolle W, Anthonsen K, Nielsen HU, Homoe P. Long-term results using LigaSure 5 mm instrument for treatment of Zenker's diverticulum. Eur Arch Otorhinolaryngol. 2017;274(4):1939–44.

41. Gonzalez N, Viola M, Costa X, Gamba A. Endoscopic treatment of Zenker's diverticulum by LigaSure scalpel. Endoscopy. 2014;46(Suppl 1 UCTN):E229–30.
42. Moreira da Silva BA, Germade A, Perez Citores L, Maestro Antolin S, Santos F, Sanchez Barranco F, et al. Endoscopic diverticulotomy using Ligasure. Gastroenterol Hepatol. 2017;40(2):80–4.
43. Noguera-Aguilar J, Dolz-Abadia C, Vilella A, Munoz-Perez JM, Canaval-Zuleta HJ, Salvatierra-Arrieta L. Transoral endoluminal approach to Zenker's diverticulum using Ligasure. Early clinical experience. Rev Esp Enferm Dig. 2014;106(2):137–41.
44. Gross ND, Cohen JI, Andersen PE. Outpatient endoscopic Zenker diverticulotomy. Laryngoscope. 2004;114(2):208–11.
45. Lang RA, Spelsberg FW, Winter H, Jauch KW, Hüttl TP. Transoral diverticulostomy with a modified Endo-Gia stapler: results after 4 years of experience. Surg Endosc. 2007;21(4):532–6. Epub 20 Dec 2006.

Flexible Endoscopic Approaches and Novel Therapy for Zenker Diverticulum

8

Ryan Law and Todd H. Baron

Introduction

There are two approaches to endoscopic cricopharyngeal myotomy for treatment of symptomatic Zenker diverticulum (ZD), one which utilizes a rigid endoscope and the other a flexible endoscope. The transoral endoscopic treatment for ZD was developed to minimize the high rate (>10%) of adverse events and mortality associated with the open surgical approach. Transoral therapy with a rigid endoscope requires significant neck extension and jaw retraction to allow passage and placement of the rigid diverticuloscope, which may not be feasible in all patients. Due to these inherent limitations of the open surgical approach and rigid endoscopic approach, a variety of techniques and methods to perform flexible endoscopic transoral cricopharyngeal myotomyc have been developed. Similar to other interventions, the flexible endoscopic technique approach aims to decrease cricopharyngeal sphincter pressure by dividing the cricopharyngeus to the apex of the diverticulum (Fig. 8.1) [1]. Treatment of ZD using a transoral flexible endoscope was initially described by Mulder and Ishioka more than 20 years ago [2, 3]. Many case series have subsequently been published establishing the outcomes of flexible endoscopic therapy [4]. Available data suggest that the safety and efficacy are comparable to the recognized outcomes of the rigid transoral endoscopic approach [5].

R. Law
Division of Gastroenterology and Hepatology, University of Michigan, Ann Arbor, MI, USA

T. H. Baron (✉)
Division of Gastroenterology and Hepatology, University of North Carolina,
Chapel Hill, NC, USA
e-mail: todd_baron@med.unc.edu

© Springer International Publishing AG, part of Springer Nature 2018
R. Scher, D. Myssiorek (eds.), *Management of Zenker and Hypopharyngeal Diverticula*, https://doi.org/10.1007/978-3-319-92156-3_8

Fig. 8.1 Endoscopic view
following complete
division of the diverticular
septum after flexible
endoscopic
cricopharyngeal myotomy

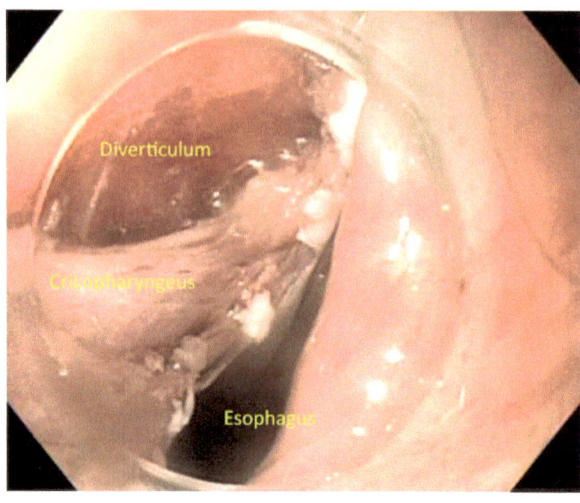

Techniques

When compared to rigid endoscopes, the fundamental advantages of the flexible
endoscopic method are due to the agility and smaller diameter of the gastroscope,
important attributes when treating patients with jaw retraction and/or limited neck
extension. Flexible endoscopic intervention may be more suitable than surgical
intervention for elderly patients or any patients with limiting medical comorbidities.
In addition, rigid endoscopy may not be possible in patients with diverticular
pouches <2 cm because it limits access of the stapler head. Contrarily, in patients
with large diverticula, the stapler may not reach the bottom of the diverticulum. In
very rare instances, patient comorbidities may limit flexible endoscopic diverticulotomy, mainly due to concerns with anesthesia. Flexible endoscopic therapy for ZD
should not be performed with conscious sedation. General anesthesia is not required;
though the risk of procedural-related aspiration is minimized by endotracheal intu-
bation, monitored anesthesia care (MAC) may be sufficient. The use of anesthesia
support is recommended due to the potential need for acute airway protection.
Available literature suggests an average of 60 minutes will be required to perform
flexible cricopharyngeal myotomy [6].

Prior to diverticulotomy, a routine upper endoscopy should be performed to identify the relationship between the ZD and true esophageal lumen. Importantly, all
remaining liquid or food debris within the ZD is evacuated. Patients are given a
single dose of broad-spectrum antibiotics prior to incision.

A soft diverticuloscope (Cook Medical, Cork, Ireland) is available outside the
United States and can be used to stabilize the septum, increase visualization, and
maintain the anatomic orientation during the incision (Fig. 8.2). This overtube was

Fig. 8.2 Zenker diverticulum overtube (AKA diverticuloscope) (Cook Medical)

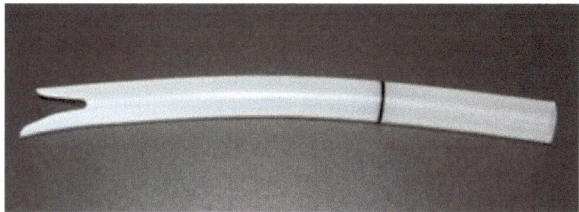

Fig. 8.3 Placement of a nasogastric tube prior to myotomy to provide orientation during the procedure. The NG tube is placed into the true esophageal lumen with the diverticular septum to the left

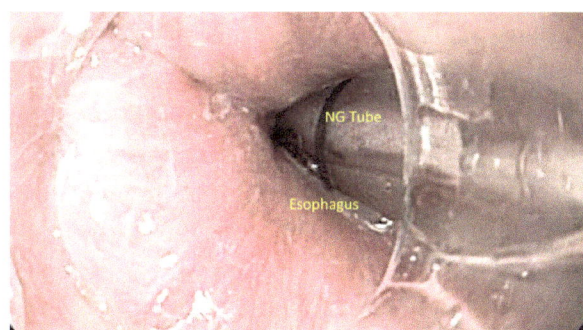

designed to mimic the rigid diverticuloscope and is loaded onto the endoscope and positioned similar to a standard overtube. The diverticuloscope has duckbill flanges at its distal end, one short flange to be seated within the ZD and one longer flange that is placed in the esophageal lumen. This construction promotes exposure and stabilization of the cricopharyngeal septum between the flanges. Positioning of the diverticuloscope may be difficult or impossible in patients with small or difficult-to-access diverticula. Transparent hoods or caps that attach to the tip of the endoscope can also be used to enhance visualization. These are readily available in most endoscopy units. Modification of a standard esophageal overtube or a clear distal attachment cap for the purpose of Zenker diverticulotomy has been previously described [7, 8].

When the soft diverticuloscope is not available, pre-procedural placement of a nasogastric (NG) tube is recommended (Fig. 8.3). The NG tube is important for two reasons. Firstly, it guides the endoscopist to the true esophageal lumen during the procedure, especially once the myotomy has commenced as the correct anatomical orientation can be easily lost. Secondly, the NG tube offers a method to supply enteral nutrition should a procedural adverse event occur, such as perforation. Blind passage of an NG tube is not recommended due to concern for inadvertent injury to the ZD. We prefer to pass a small caliber endoscope transnasally followed by guidewire placement into the stomach. The endoscope is then withdrawn leaving the guidewire in place. A small hole is made in the distal tip of the NG tube using an 18G needle. The NG tube is passed over the guidewire, and the NG tube is positioned in the stomach. This method negates the need for oral-to-nasal transfer of the guidewire.

Several methods to incise the cricopharyngeus muscle have been described, including use of endoscopic submucosal dissection (ESD) techniques, submucosal tunneling, and creation of a wedge-shaped incision [9, 10]. The cricopharyngeus muscle (septum) is divided using needle knives designed for pancreaticobiliary use or other electrocautery-enhanced accessories designed for ESD, such as a hook knife (Olympus America, Center Valley, PA) (Fig. 8.4) [11]. Other through-the-scope tools which can be used to divide the septum include argon plasma coagulation, monopolar and bipolar forceps, and endoscopic scissor forceps (stag beetle [SB] knife [Olympus America], Clutch Cutter [Fujifilm Europe, Dusseldorf, Germany]) (Fig. 8.5). We most frequently use the hook knife and utilize standard sphincterotomy settings (Endocut I, effect 2) on our electrosurgical generator. The use of harmonic scalpels and other surgical stapling devices has been described and requires passage of a flexible endoscope alongside the device as these devices are too large to pass through the

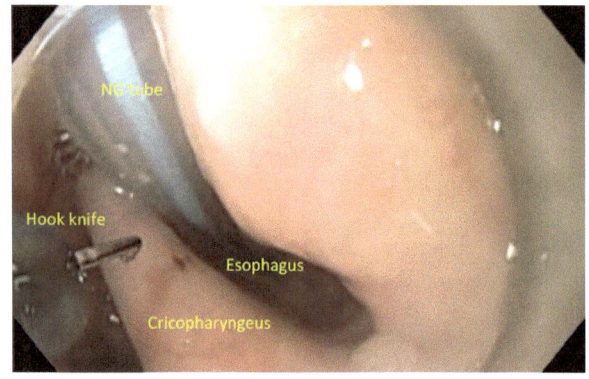

Fig. 8.4 Hook knife (Olympus America) used to perform cricopharyngeal myotomy. The hook tip allows for tissue capture and stability during incision

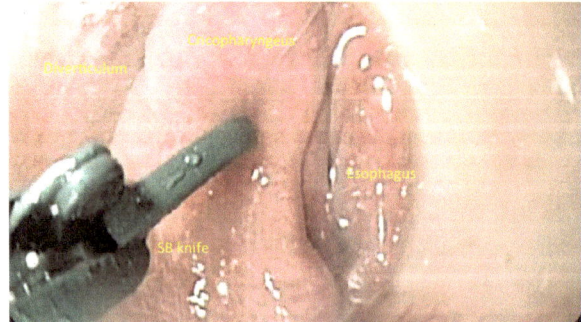

Fig. 8.5 SB knife (Olympus America) used to perform cricopharyngeal myotomy. The scissorlike shape allows for division of the septum while maintaining control of the intended cutting path

flexible endoscope working channel [12–16]. Following complete division of the cricopharyngeus, many endoscopists opt to place through-the-scope endoscopic clips at the diverticular apex with the goal of preventing delayed perforation. The optimal cutting device and technique remain unclear.

Perioperative Care

There is no consensus on routine use of pre-procedural or post-procedural antibiotics, hospital admission, diet, and follow-up imaging studies. Following the procedure, strong consideration should be given to observing the patient in the hospital for overnight observation, especially if the procedure was complicated by intraprocedural bleeding and/or possible perforation or if the patient has traveled from a distance. An esophagram using water-soluble contrast medium should be performed immediately in patients with suspected perforation. Local patients or those with uncomplicated procedures can be discharged home with follow-up plan in place. A routine follow-up esophagram should be obtained to evaluate for a residual septum. Virtually all patients will have post-procedural throat pain, which may require short-term narcotic analgesics. Some endoscopists recommend continuation of oral antibiotic therapy for 5 days after the procedure. We routinely allow peroral intake of liquids shortly after the procedure in the absence of suspected adverse events. The diet is slowly advanced as tolerated. A recommended diet is clear liquids for 24 h, followed by full liquids for 24 h, and then slowly advance to tolerance thereafter.

Results

Available data show that >90% of patients will have durable symptom relief following diverticulotomy using the flexible endoscopic approach [17]. Manometric studies have demonstrated efficacy in reducing UES pressure after flexible endoscopic cricopharyngeal myotomy [1]. Available data suggest that symptom relief can be provided in one to two procedures with a high rate of clinical improvement and low rate of persistence on radiography [4]. Recurrence or persistence of clinical symptoms occurs in 11% and may be related to persistence of cricopharyngeus musculature [17]; however, no consensus definition of post-intervention clinical success exists. In our opinion, clinical success should be based solely on improvement in clinical symptoms on a patient-by-patient basis. Radiographic or endoscopic findings of a refractory septum and/or residual diverticulum do not correlate with symptom persistence or recurrence after intervention. It should be noted that many of the currently available case series provide little to no post-intervention clinical follow-up.

Adverse Events

The median adverse event rate following flexible endoscopic therapy is approximately 11% (range 0–36%), based on currently available literature [17]. Postprocedural throat pain is nearly uniform and may require narcotic analgesics, usually for up to 72 h. Bleeding is the most common intraprocedural event occurring in <5% cases [4]. This is generally self-limited during the procedure; however, persistent oozing during the procedure may require endoscopic control using routine hemostasis intervention (i.e., electrocautery devices, endoclip placement, epinephrine injection). A recent meta-analysis by Ishaq et al. found the rate of perforation to be 6.5% [17]. A microperforation can manifest as subcutaneous emphysema but is frequently uncomplicated. Air tracking within the submucosal plane in the absence of a perforation may also be seen [18]. Following the procedure, patients should be followed closely, though subcutaneous emphysema in an asymptomatic patient should not necessitate surgical intervention. The use of carbon dioxide for insufflation in all patients undergoing Zenker therapy remains the current standard of care and may minimize adverse events. The most feared adverse event is perforation into the mediastinum, a relatively uncommon adverse event during flexible endoscopic intervention when performed by experienced therapeutic endoscopists. Available data demonstrate a median perforation/leak rate of 4%, regardless whether or not endoscopic clips are placed at the diverticular apex following myotomy [19, 20]. Concern for a frank mediastinal perforation should prompt an oral contrast study with gastrografin to identify potential sites of extravasation. Otherwise, a CT scan of the neck and chest with administration of oral contrast could also be considered.

Training in Flexible Endoscopic Cricopharyngeal Myotomy

Treatment of ZD with the flexible endoscopic approach should only be performed by expert therapeutic endoscopists with training in advanced endoscopy after careful consideration of the risks and benefits of the procedure. The relative rarity of patients with ZD requiring flexible endoscopic intervention is not conducive for inexperienced endoscopists to safely perform this procedure. Expertise in the use of various electrocautery devices is needed when performing Zenker diverticulotomy. Many techniques and accessories used during flexible endoscopic cricopharyngeal myotomy were originally designed for endoscopic submucosal dissection (ESD) and peroral endoscopic myotomy (POEM) [6]. Therapeutic endoscopists with advanced training in ESD/POEM may be best prepared to implement transoral flexible endoscopic therapy of Zenker diverticulum.

Preclinical training using an animal model is recommended, if available. Animal training allows the endoscopist to gain familiarity with the procedure, such as the distinctive endoscopic view, gastroscope stability in the proximal esophagus, and correct identification of esophageal wall layers during incision. A porcine animal model has been previously described in the literature [21]. Pigs are an ideal model for flexible endoscopic cricopharyngeal myotomy as their normal anatomic pharyngeal pouch closely resembles a ZD.

Conclusions

The principle of endoscopic cricopharyngeal incision as a treatment of symptomatic ZD has remained unchanged for decades. Rigid transoral endoscopic intervention remains the most common treatment modality. Available data on the flexible endoscopic approach have demonstrated equivalent efficacy when compared to the rigid endoscopic approach, with acceptable adverse event rates. The ongoing development of flexible endoscopic treatments allows skilled endoscopists the opportunity to effectively and safely treat patients with symptomatic ZD.

References

1. Ishioka S, Felix VN, Sakai P, et al. Manometric study of the upper esophageal sphincter before and after endoscopic management of Zenker's diverticulum. Hepatogastroenterology. 1995;42:628–32.
2. Ishioka S, Sakai P, Maluf Filho F, et al. Endoscopic incision of Zenker's diverticula. Endoscopy. 1995;27:433–7.
3. Mulder CJ, den Hartog G, Robijn RJ, et al. Flexible endoscopic treatment of Zenker's diverticulum: a new approach. Endoscopy. 1995;27:438–42.
4. Law R, Katzka DA, Baron TH. Zenker's diverticulum. Clin Gastroenterol Hepatol. 2014;12:1773–82; quiz e111–2.
5. Repici A, Pagano N, Fumagalli U, et al. Transoral treatment of Zenker diverticulum: flexible endoscopy versus endoscopic stapling. A retrospective comparison of outcomes. Dis Esophagus. 2011;24:235–9.
6. Katzka DA, Baron TH. Transoral flexible endoscopic therapy of Zenker's diverticulum: is it time for gastroenterologists to stick their necks out? Gastrointest Endosc. 2013;77:708–10.
7. Seaman DL, de la Mora Levy J, Gostout CJ, et al. A new device to simplify flexible endoscopic treatment of Zenker's diverticulum. Gastrointest Endosc. 2008;67:112–5.
8. Tang SJ. Flexible endoscopic Zenker's diverticulotomy: approach that involves thinking outside the box (with videos). Surg Endosc. 2014;28:1355–9.
9. Kedia P, Fukami N, Kumta NA, et al. A novel method to perform endoscopic myotomy for Zenker's diverticulum using submucosal dissection techniques. Endoscopy. 2014;46: 1119–21.
10. Li QL, Chen WF, Zhang XC, et al. Submucosal tunneling endoscopic septum division: a novel technique for treating Zenker's diverticulum. Gastroenterology. 2016;151:1071–4.
11. Halland M, Grooteman KV, Baron TH. Flexible endosopic management of Zenker's diverticulum: characteristics and outcomes of 52 cases at a tertiary referral center. Dis Esophagus. 2016;29:273–7.
12. Rieder E, Martinec DV, Dunst CM, et al. Flexible endoscopic Zenkers diverticulotomy with a novel bipolar forceps: a pilot study and comparison with needleknife dissection. Surg Endosc. 2011;25:3273–8.
13. Neumann H, Loffler S, Rieger S, et al. Endoscopic therapy of Zenker's diverticulum using a novel endoscopic scissor – the Clutch Cutter device. Endoscopy. 2015;47(Suppl 1 UCTN):E430–1.
14. Goelder SK, Brueckner J, Messmann H. Endoscopic treatment of Zenker's diverticulum with the stag beetle knife (sb knife) - feasibility and follow-up. Scand J Gastroenterol. 2016;51:1155–8.

15. Adam SI, Paskhover B, Sasaki CT. Laser versus stapler: outcomes in endoscopic repair of Zenker diverticulum. Laryngoscope. 2012;122:1961–6.
16. Heinrich H, Bauerfeind P. Endoscopic treatment of Zenker's diverticulum using a hook knife. Endoscopy. 2009;41(Suppl 2):E311–2.
17. Ishaq S, Hassan C, Antonello A, et al. Flexible endoscopic treatment for Zenker's diverticulum: a systematic review and meta-analysis. Gastrointest Endosc. 2016;83:1076–1089.e5.
18. Baron TH, Wong Kee Song LM, Zielinski MD, et al. A comprehensive approach to the management of acute endoscopic perforations (with videos). Gastrointest Endosc. 2012;76:838–59.
19. Dzeletovic I, Ekbom DC, Baron TH. Flexible endoscopic and surgical management of Zenker's diverticulum. Expert Rev Gastroenterol Hepatol. 2012;6:449–65; quiz 466.
20. Sakai P. Endoscopic myotomy of Zenker's diverticulum: lessons from 3 decades of experience. Gastrointest Endosc. 2016;83:774–5.
21. Seaman DL, de la Mora Levy J, Gostout CJ, et al. An animal training model for endoscopic treatment of Zenker's diverticulum. Gastrointest Endosc. 2007;65:1050–3.

Mark A. Fritz, Christopher M. Johnson,
and Gregory N. Postma

Introduction

Zenker diverticulum (ZD) is by far and away the most common hypopharyngeal or esophageal diverticulum found in humans. It has an estimated prevalence of 0.01–0.11% in the population [1]. The first successful reported surgical procedure to remove ZD was in 1886 by Wheeler. While there is a good amount of literature about ZD, due to the much lower prevalence of non-Zenker diverticula (nZD), there are no large epidemiological reports and very little data beyond case reports in the literature to describe them.

Pharyngeal and esophageal diverticula can be classified by location along the digestive tract, such as within the hypopharynx, mid-thoracic, or epiphrenic regions [2]. Additionally, due to their different pathophysiology, they can be further broken down into either pulsion or traction diverticula (TD) and either true or false diverticula. Pulsion diverticula by definition herniate through a weakness in the outer muscular wall due to an increased intraluminal pressure and are hence typically considered false diverticula due to the presence of only mucosa and submucosa within the wall of the pouch. TD form from external tethering of the pharynx or esophagus to an adjacent inflammatory nidus and typically consist of all three layers of mucosa, submucosa, and outer muscular layers making it a true diverticulum. The most common diverticulum, the ZD, is classified as a hypopharyngeal, pulsion, false diverticulum. Pulsion diverticula typically form in the hypopharyngeal and epiphrenic regions due to either cricopharyngeus (CP) dysfunction or lower

M. A. Fritz (✉)
Department of Otolaryngology—Head and Neck Surgery, University of Kentucky,
Lexington, KY, USA

C. M. Johnson
Department of Otolaryngology, Naval Medical Center, San Diego, CA, USA

G. N. Postma
Department of Otolaryngology—Head and Neck Surgery, Medical College
of Georgia at Augusta University, Augusta, GA, USA

© Springer International Publishing AG, part of Springer Nature 2018
R. Scher, D. Myssiorek (eds.), *Management of Zenker and Hypopharyngeal Diverticula*, https://doi.org/10.1007/978-3-319-92156-3_9

esophageal sphincter dysfunction leading to increased intraluminal pressures. TD on the other hand are typically found in the mid-thoracic region due to a classical association with hilar lymphadenopathy from such conditions as neoplasia, tuberculosis, or fungal infections.

This chapter will describe most of the exceptions to the classical descriptions and describe the pathophysiology for several other types of diverticula. While ZD is a pulsion type diverticulum that occurs above the CP muscle, Laimer and Killian-Jamieson diverticula are also thought to be pulsion diverticula, but they originate below the CP. Additionally,)TD can occur outside the typical mid-thoracic region as evidenced by more and more reports over the last few decades of iatrogenic diverticula thought to be directly related to anterior approaches to the cervical spine. The important difference for these other diverticula is that they typically cannot be treated through endoscopic means which is becoming the preferred means at some institutions for treatment of the more common ZD. Additionally, a standard barium esophagram will sometimes be unable to make the distinction between these entities, so prior knowledge to help with surgical consent and planning is critical.

There are three anatomical areas of weakness in the pharyngeal musculature through which pulsion diverticula protrude (Fig. 9.1). Killian's triangle represents an area between the inferior constrictor muscles above and the CP more caudally. ZD herniate through this area of weakness classically described as being concurrent with CP muscle dysfunction which builds the pressure required to create the outpouching. The false ZD then protrudes posteriorly into the retropharyngeal space and nearly all extend slightly left. If the pouch is very large, it can bulge out even further laterally into the visceral space.

The Killian-Jamieson area sits below the CP muscle laterally and represents the spot where the recurrent laryngeal nerve (RLN) enters the larynx. Killian-Jamieson

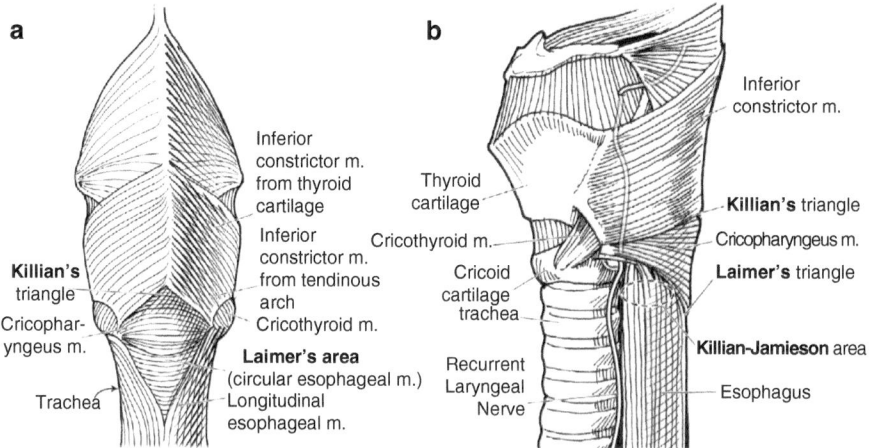

Fig. 9.1 (a) Left shows the posterior view of the pharyngoesophagus. (b) Shows the lateral view. Both highlight the Killian's triangle, Laimer's triangle, and the Killian-Jamieson area where ZD, KJD, and LD arise (Reprinted with permission from Elsevier [2])

diverticula (KJD) originate in this region. In 1983, the first large report on KJD was published, including 13 individual cases [3]. KJD are considered pulsion diverticula and are almost exclusively found on the left side, except where seen bilaterally in a few patients. Due to this lateral location and the fact that the area of dehiscence is related to the entrance of the RLN, the nerve is especially at risk during surgery. Accordingly, while there are endoscopic reports of treating KJD [4, 5], the open cervical approach is typically performed to minimize possible damage to the RLN [6]. There have been reports of this diverticulum being coincident with a ZD [7].

Laimer's triangle or the Laimer-Haeckerman area of weakness sits in a triangular area below the cricopharyngeus and between the divergent longitudinal muscle fibers of the proximal esophagus where only the circular fibers of the esophagus are present. This area is where the Laimer diverticulum (LD) arises. Of those seen, most are described as true diverticula. Boysen et al. depicted a case of a coinciding LD along with a ZD [8]. All in all, there have been only a handful of reports in the literature about LD [8–11]. Esophageal dysmotility is thought to be the underlying causation for the development of this diverticulum and is hence considered pulsion in origin [10].

While ZD, KJD, and LD are all pulsion diverticula and all)have distinct anatomical locations due to muscular areas of weakness, iatrogenic or infectious TD can occur virtually anywhere dependent upon where the inflammatory source is located. Figure 9.2 depicts all of these diverticula in the relationships to the hypopharyngeal musculature. Classically, these occurred due to scarring or tethering of the esophageal or hypopharyngeal musculature to the surrounding tissue. However, in 1991, there was a first report of a hypopharyngeal TD) that was associated with a history of an anterior approach to the cervical spine [12]. While there are only a few cases reported in the literature associated with these anterior approaches, it has been postulated by some that this number may rise given the popularity of the approach among spine surgeons [13]. Additionally, these TD might be difficult to spot as they may mimic ZD in appearance, especially around the region of C4–C7, in all respects except for the presence of anterior spinal hardware.

Diagnosis

The clinical presentation for all of these diverticula is virtually identical. Solid food dysphagia and more specifically regurgitation are the primary presenting symptoms of patients with these hypopharyngeal diverticula. TD are classically associated with prior anterior cervical spine surgery, esophageal perforation, or infection, so a full history is critical to elucidating the type of hypopharyngeal diverticulum involved.

The most useful diagnostic tool for identifying hypopharyngeal diverticula is a barium esophagram or modified barium swallow. Either of these should readily identify a diverticulum described above. The most important part of the study is identification of the actual CP muscle to determine its relationship to the diverticulum. In some difficult cases, a frame-by-frame review is needed. As discussed above, the

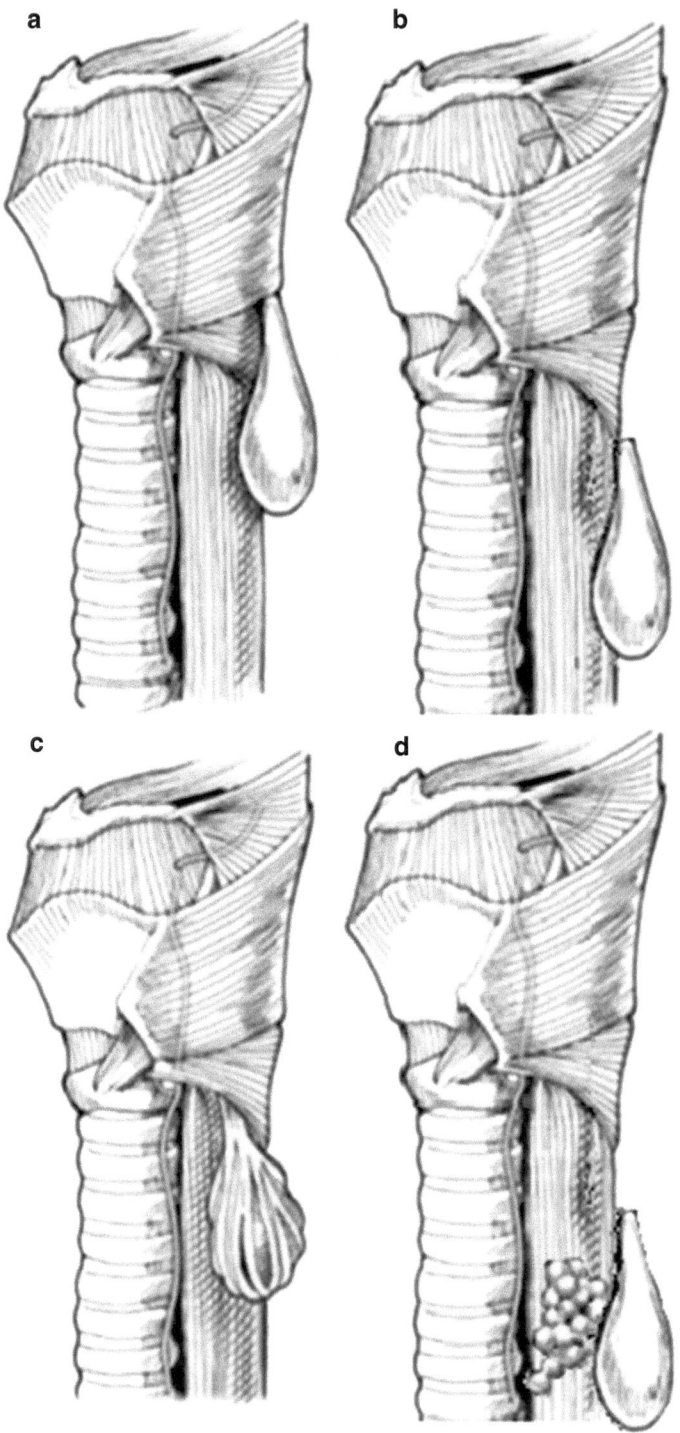

Fig. 9.2 These drawings depict the relationship of the musculature where the various diverticula arise. They consist of ZD (**a**), KJD (**b**), LD (**c**), and traction (**d**) (Reprinted with permission from Elsevier [2])

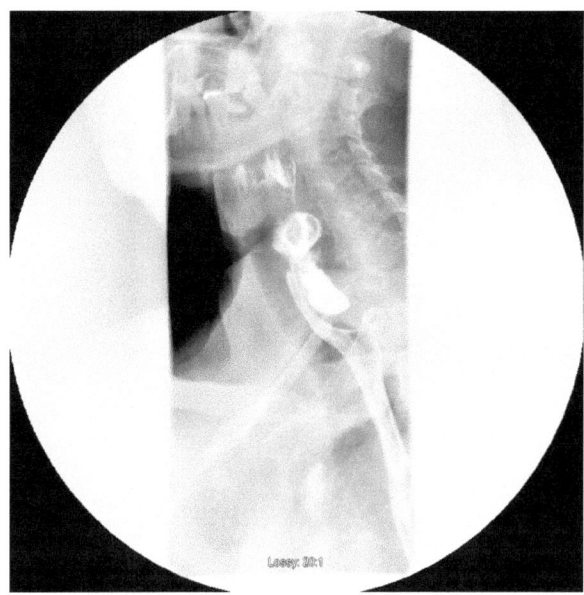

Fig. 9.3 Lateral view of a barium swallow showing a ZD. Typically contrast will get stuck in the pouch and remain even after the esophageal bolus has passed by. It will often be of slightly different density

ZD will present above the CP muscle on lateral view (Fig. 9.3), but the LD and KJD will present below the CP. KJD can also show a similar-looking pouch on anterior view (Fig. 9.4). As the radiographic image can also show cervical hardware with ease, this element of their history and the relationship to the pouch should be readily apparent as well at this stage. However, sometimes it is difficult or impossible to tell the relationship to the CP muscle without direct or endoscopic visualization either prior to or at the time of surgery.

Pulsion diverticula are classically associated with an increased intraluminal pressure because of CP dysfunction or underlying esophageal dysmotility. In this respect, high-resolution esophageal manometry can reveal useful information prior to any surgical intervention. While this is not essential to the management, it may help guide surgical planning due to its ability to distinguish between pulsion and TD.

Treatment

There are essentially two surgical options for the treatment of hypopharyngeal diverticula: open and endoscopic. The first open diverticulectomy was reported in the late 1880s by Wheeler. Mosher in 1914 reported the first endoscopic treatment of a ZD. However, this was abandoned by Mosher himself due to unacceptable mortality presumably from mediastinitis. In 1960, endoscopic treatment started becoming more feasible with the use of the carbon dioxide laser and subsequently

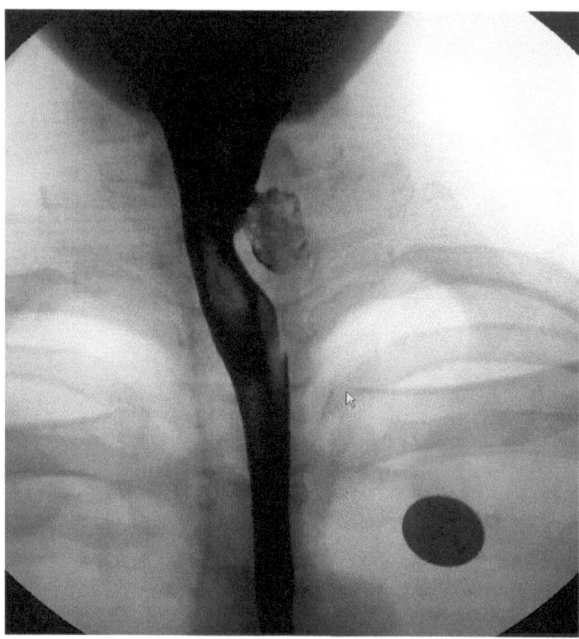

Fig. 9.4 Anteroposterior view of the esophagus and KJD during a barium swallow. The appearance mimics a barium swallow for ZD but instead shows a bar-like structure in A–P presentation

started gaining widespread use in the 1990s with the introduction of the endoscopic stapler technique (endoscopic staple-assisted diverticulostomy). While the endoscopic approach has become popular for treatment of ZD, the endoscopic treatment of other hypopharyngeal diverticula has not been well established. As stated previously, an open approach is favored for KJD due to the intimate association with the RLN next to the pouch. New flexible endoscopic approaches to the diverticula that are in the literature utilizing the esophagogastroduodenoscope are not advocated for these pouches as they put the RLN at risk for injury. Moreover, Ba and colleagues in their description of a series of TD postulated that thick scarring of the diverticular wall could prohibit endoscopic stapling altogether [14].

Endoscopic exposure of a ZD pouch is difficult and requires skill and favorable anatomy, but exposure below the cricopharyngeus is challenging at best. However, the endoscopic exposure of these diverticula is still often attempted at first because of decreased operative time, decreased pain, and faster return to oral diet that is thought to result with endoscopic management. When an iatrogenic hypopharyngeal TD is treated, removal of the cervical spinal hardware is sometimes required, which necessitates preoperative planning with a spine surgeon. An open approach would obviously be more ideal for this removal of hardware and would therefore grant the exposure needed for the diverticulectomy.

For the endoscopic approach, a Weerda distending diverticuloscope (Storz, Goleta, CA) is used to attempt to expose the pouch transorally. An attempt is made to place one tine of the scope in the esophagus and one in the pouch. This is successful in roughly 80–90% of patients in our practice. However, exposure is rarely successful below the cricopharyngeus which represent most non-Zenker diverticula. For this reason, we prefer to obtain surgical consent for endoscopic and open approaches to the diverticulum prior to surgery.

Even if an open approach is planned, an endoscopic exposure is typically attempted in order to pack the diverticulum with gauze and directly place an esophageal dilator that would assist in the identification of the esophagus through the open approach. Alternatively, it is our practice to use the trans-nasal esophagoscope to help with the identification of the esophagus from the open approach but also provide illumination from inside the pouch and insufflate the pouch with air to allow better visualization and easier dissection [15]. With the open approach, it is also our practice to give 24 h of intravenous antibiotics (clindamycin or ampicillin/sulbactam) with the first dose given perioperatively.

In the open approach, a 5 cm horizontal skin incision is made at the level of the inferior border of the thyroid cartilage slightly lateral to the midline. The anterior-posterior view of the barium study should be reviewed just before the skin incision to ensure the correct side. In most cases, diverticula will extend either posteriorly or to the left within the visceral space. Subplatysmal flaps are raised superiorly and inferiorly. The anterior border of the sternocleidomastoid muscle is delineated, and the omohyoid muscle is identified. Then the lateral edge of the infrahyoid strap muscles and the laryngotracheal complex are identified. Dissection then proceeds between the laryngotracheal complex and the carotid sheath toward the retropharynx. The omohyoid muscle can be incised to improve access, but is not always necessary. The laryngotracheal complex is retracted by placing a blunt double-prong skin retractor on the posterior edge of the thyroid cartilage to further expose the diverticulum and surrounding tissue. Palpation of the esophageal dilator, gauze packing, or alternatively visualization of the light and air insufflation from the transnasal esophagoscope is useful at this stage to confirm identification of the esophagus and the pouch. Once this pouch is identified, it is dissected free of the surrounding tissue until the neck is clearly defined, taking care as the RLN passes near this area. In the case of the KJD, the RLN is identified and carefully freed from the diverticular pouch. It is at this time that any lymphadenopathy, signs of infection, scarring, or prior injury is assessed, especially if a TD is suspected. If the pouch is near and above the CP muscle, then a CP myotomy is performed. A linear stapler is then brought into the surgical bed and firstly squeezed tight while assessing the patency of the esophageal narrowing before fully excising the pouch along the staple line. After the pouch is excised, the wound bed can be filled with saline and the transnasal esophagoscope used to insufflate air into the esophagus to perform a leak test. If no leak is identified, the incision is then closed in layers (a surgical drain may be used per surgeon preference), and the procedure is completed with the patient being nothing by mouth for the rest of that day and starting on clear liquids and advancing quickly the next morning if there is no fever, tachycardia, chest pain, or neck crepitus.

Conclusion

While non-Zenker hypopharyngeal diverticula are considerably rarer in incidence, their management is inherently different from the more common ZD. Even though the diagnosis of most hypopharyngeal pouches is made using barium esophagography, identification of these less common diverticula is difficult to make using radiographic studies alone unless clinical suspicion is very high. Therefore, surgeons should be familiar with these diverticula other than ZD and plan their patient's surgery accordingly.

References

1. Watemberg S, Landau O, Avrahami R. Zenker's diverticulum: reappraisal. Am J Gastroenterol. 1996;91:1494–8.
2. Johnson CM, Postma GN. Not all pharyngeal pouches are created equal: management of "non-Zenker" hypopharyngeal diverticula. Oper Tech Otolaryngol Head Neck Surg. 2016;27:80–5.
3. Ekberg O, Nylander G. Lateral diverticula from the pharyngo-esophageal junction area. Radiology. 1983;146:117–22.
4. Tang SJ, Tang L, Chen E, Myers LL. Flexible endoscopic Killian-Jamieson diverticulotomy and literature review (with video). Gastrointest Endosc. 2008;68:790–3.
5. Lee CK, Chung IK, Park JY, Lee TH, Lee SH, Park SH, Kim HS, Kim SJ. Endoscopic diverticulotomy with an isolated-tip needle-knife papillotome (Iso-Tome) and a fitted overtube for the treatment of a Killian-Jamieson diverticulum. World J Gastroenterol. 2008;14:6589–92.
6. Undavia S, Anand SM, Jacobson AS. Killian-Jamieson diverticulum. Laryngoscope. 2013;123:414–7.
7. Stewart KE, Smith DRK, Woolley SL. Simultaneously occurring Zenker's diverticulum and Killian–Jamieson diverticulum: case report and literature review. J Laryngol Otol. 2017;131:661–6.
8. Boysen M, Aasen S, Lotveit T, Bakka A. Two simultaneously occurring hypopharyngo-oesophageal diverticula. J Laryngol Otol. 1993;107:49–50.
9. Kobayashi M, Sawada T, Deguchi M, Lin S, Okada D, Ohe H, et al. A case of diverticulum originating from the Laimer's triangle. Geka Shinryou. 1993;36:888–92.
10. Kumoi K, Ohtsuki N, Teramoto Y. Pharyngo-esophageal diverticulum arising from Laimer's triangle. Eur Arch Otorhinolaryngol. 2001;258:184–7.
11. Nguyen D, Moslemi M, Rawashdeh B, Meyer M, Garagozlo C. Laimer's diverticulum, a rare true diverticulum inferior to the cricopharyngeus: report of a case and review of the literature. J Clin Case Rep. 2014;4:2.
12. Goffart Y, Lenelle J, Moreau P, Boverie J. Traction diverticulum of the hypopharynx following anterior cervical spine surgery:case report and review. Ann Otol Rhinol Laryngol. 1991;100:852–5.
13. Allis TJ, Grant NN, Davidson BJ. Hypopharyngeal diverticulum formation following anterior discectomy and fusion: case series. Ear Nose Throat J. 2010;89:E4–9.
14. Alyssa MB, LoTempio MM, Wang MB. Pharyngeal diverticulum as a sequela of anterior cervical fusion. Otolaryngol Head Neck Surg. 2004;131:P256–P7.
15. Segel J HR, Postma GN. The utility of flexible esophagoscopy during endoscopic and open Zenker's surgery. In: Fall voice conference, San Antonio, TX; 2014.

Index

© Springer International Publishing AG, part of Springer Nature 2018
R. Scher, D. Myssiorek (eds.), *Management of Zenker and Hypopharyngeal
Diverticula*, https://doi.org/10.1007/978-3-319-92156-3